MEASUREMENTS IN RADIOLOGY
Made Easy®

System requirement:

- **Windows XP or above**
- **Power DVD player (Software)**
- **Windows media player 11.0 version or above (Software)**

Accompanying Interactive Photo CD ROM is playable only in Computer and not in DVD player.

Kindly wait for few seconds for DVD to autorun. If it does not autorun then please do the following:

- Click on my computer

- Click the **CD/DVD drive** and after opening the drive, kindly double click the file **Jaypee**

MEASUREMENTS IN RADIOLOGY
Made Easy®

Vineet Wadhwa
MBBS DMRD OSGH (Singapore)
FRHS FAGE FWSIM (USA) MIRIA MECR
Radiologist, Delhi State Cancer Institute
Dilshad Garden, Delhi, India
Premier Institute of Delhi Government for Oncology
Formerly Registrar, Department of Radiodiagnosis
St Stephen's Hospital, Tis Hazari, New Delhi, India
Email: *wadhwa39@yahoo.co.in*

Forewords
Kishore V Hegde
Anuradha Sural
Umesh K

JAYPEE BROTHERS MEDICAL PUBLISHERS (P) LTD

New Delhi • St Louis • Panama City • London

Published by

Jaypee Brothers Medical Publishers (P) Ltd

Corporate Office

4838/24, Ansari Road, Daryaganj, **New Delhi** 110 002, India
Phone: +91-11-43574357, Fax: +91-11-43574314

Offices in India

- **Ahmedabad,** e-mail: ahmedabad@jaypeebrothers.com
- **Bengaluru,** e-mail: bangalore@jaypeebrothers.com
- **Chennai,** e-mail: chennai@jaypeebrothers.com
- **Delhi,** e-mail: jaypee@jaypeebrothers.com
- **Hyderabad,** e-mail: hyderabad@jaypeebrothers.com
- **Kochi,** e-mail: kochi@jaypeebrothers.com
- **Kolkata,** e-mail: kolkata@jaypeebrothers.com
- **Lucknow,** e-mail: lucknow@jaypeebrothers.com
- **Mumbai,** e-mail: mumbai@jaypeebrothers.com
- **Nagpur,** e-mail: nagpur@jaypeebrothers.com

Overseas Offices

- **North America Office, USA,** Ph: 001-636-6279734
  e-mail: jaypee@jaypeebrothers.com, anjulav@jaypeebrothers.com
- **Central America Office, Panama City, Panama**
  Ph: 001-507-317-0160 e-mail: cservice@jphmedical.com,
  Website: www.jphmedical.com
- **Europe Office, UK,** Ph: +44 (0) 2031708910
  e-mail: info@jpmedpub.com

Measurements in Radiology Made Easy®

© 2011, Jaypee Brothers Medical Publishers

First Edition: 2011

ISBN 978-93-5025-264-2

Typeset at JPBMP typesetting unit

Printed at Rajkamal Electric Press, Plot No. 2, Phase-IV, Kundli, Haryana.

Dedicated to

Shri Morari Bapu

and

My grandparents
Late Shri Hakim Jamman Dass Wadhwa
and Late Smt Chandni Bai Wadhwa

Foreword

It gives me great sense of pride in writing foreword for this book and congratulate my student Dr Vineet Wadhwa on this first of its kind compilation in radiology.

In this book, he has compiled a comprehensive list of measurements covering all the systems from central nervous system (CNS) to ENT including embryological criteria. This book will be handy not only in times of uncertainty in aiding diagnosis but also as a rapid reckoner. The accurate measurements have also been updated from the latest journals, keeping abreast of the latest developments. The detailed listing makes it useful also for differential diagnosis.

I wish him greater success in all his future endeavors. He is also the author of another famous book on clinical methods. I am sure this book on measurements will be popular and supporting not only among radiologists but also among all our colleagues of medicine.

Wishing him all the success...

Kishore V Hegde
Professor and Head
Department of Radiology
Narayana Medical College
Nellore, Andhra Pradesh
India

Foreword

I consider it a privilege to contribute a foreword to this book which is the product of Dr Vineet's hard work. It presents well-organized various measurements used in radiology, data which every radiologist should know. Normal measurements with differential diagnosis of altered measurements are also mentioned.

Presented in an easy-to-carry pocket book size, with simple language and diagrams, the book is a storehouse of useful information, with separate chapters on age determination, Hounsfield unit values and staging of various pathologies.

I feel it will be a useful book, not only for radiology residents but also for practitioners.

I congratulate him on his laudable effort.

Anuradha Sural
Consultant Radiologist
Department of Radiodiagnosis
St Stephen's Hospital, New Delhi
India

Foreword

It gives me immense pleasure to give foreword for my student Dr Vineet Wadhwa whom I know since his post-graduation days.

Radiology is the fastest advancing branch of medical sciences. It plays an important role in diagnosis of various pathologies. This book is an excellent compilation of various measurements used in radiology, arranged in systematic way. It also has separate chapters on age determination, rules in radiology, MR spectroscopy, Hounsfield unit values, which are very useful for our daily practice.

It has come out well, accept my congratulations...

Umesh K
Professor and Head
Sri Devaraj Urs Medical College
Kolar, Karnataka
India

Preface

Radiology though being restricted to only analyzing images, carries a greater depth to it in encompassing all the forms and fields of medicine from embryology, pathology to treatment and its response. The importance of radiology in the present set-up is very high and no patient work-up is complete without a radiological investigation.

Quantitative and qualitative perspectives have always been the two sides of a coin in radiology. Both have been synergistic to each other in not only identifying the lesion, characterizing it but also in guiding effective planning of management, its execution and follow-up. The role of measurements so plays a more integral part at all these levels. Measurements also provide a distinct sense of accuracy and specificity in aiding diagnosis.

The experience of taking various measurements in radiology during my postgraduate days made me realize the need for handbook in simple, concise, tabular and diagrammatic format to facilitate the easy and fast reporting of various cases by radiologists.

Data contained in this book is compiled from various standard radiology textbooks (refer Bibliography), journals and Internet over the years since my postgraduate days, this will be companion to standard textbooks. I sincerely hope that this book will help all the radiologists in their day-to-day practice.

I have taken utmost care in preparing the book *To err is human*, so critical appraisal of the book and suggestions for further improvements from radiologists are welcome.

Vineet Wadhwa

Acknowledgments

I am thankful to almighty God for his blessings, divine presence and masterly guidance which helps me to fulfill all goals. I am grateful to my family for their love, understanding, dedication, sacrifice, guidance and encouragement during all spheres of life. My parents Dr SP Wadhwa, Smt Santosh Wadhwa, my brother Dr Puneet, my sister-in-law Dr Shivani, my niece Aanya, my fiancée Dr Lalita, my in-laws Dr MD Naidu, Dr Suseela Naidu.

My sincere thanks to all my teachers in college and special thanks to Dr Umesh K (Professor and Head, Sri Devaraj Urs Medical College, Kolar, Karnataka, India), Professor Patabi Raman V, Professor Poornima Hegde, Dr Vinay NVP, Dr Anil Saklecha, Dr Navin M, Dr Sudhindra, Dr Bashir, Dr Ashwathnarayana.

Also thanks to Dr Nitin Parkhe, Dr Anuradha Sural, Dr Elshieba Patras, Dr Chauhan (St Stephen's Hospital, Delhi), Dr Grover (Director, Delhi State Cancer Institute).

My heartful thanks to Dr YS Deepak, Dr Vikas Kumar Sharma, Dr Timanna, Dr Jaiger, Dr Abhishek Khurana for supporting, encouraging and giving valuable suggestions during the course of the book.

I am also thankful to Dr Deepak Pahwa, Dr Hanu Tej, Dr Labh Chand Jain, Dr Apar Jindal, Dr Tarun Bali, Dr Ashish Pandey, Dr Vishal Batra, Dr Sankalan Saha, Dr Sameer Sethi, Dr Prashant Gupta, Dr Sandeep Ahuja, Dr Suresha, Dr Suresh Babu, Dr Praveen Jain, Dr Prateek Joshi, Dr Akshay Patel, Dr Ashwin Kumar, Dr Manjunath Abbigeri, Dr Wisal, Dr Shadab, Dr Gautam Jain, Dr Abhishek

XVI **MEASUREMENTS IN RADIOLOGY MADE EASY**

Fredrick, Dr Sameer Upadhyay, Dr Sahil, Dr Farhan Aijaz,
Dr Ankur Gupta, Dr Ankush, Dr Atul, Dr Deepak Mangla,
Dr Abhishek Jaiswal, Dr Kanchan, Dr Yasrab Khan,
Dr Yanya (Delhi State Cancer Institute), Dr Rajesh Pahwa,
Dr Parvez, Dr KK Mishra, Dr Vivek, Dr Gaurav Mehta,
Dr Ayan, Dr Atik Ahmed, Dr Harsha, Dr Nikhil Goyal,
Dr Vinod Reddy, Dr Sriram V, Mahipal Chaudhary,
Himanshu Gandhi, Ashish Gandhi, Vikas Kathuria,
Paras Ahuja.

I am grateful to Dr Umesh K, Dr Anuradha Sural and
Dr Kishore V Hegde for their valuable forewords; last but
not least M/s Jaypee Brothers Medical Publishers (P) Ltd,
New Delhi for accepting my work for publication.

Contents

Chapter 1

Gastrointestinal System

ANATOMY OF GASTROESOPHAGEAL JUNCTION (FIG. 1.1)

B ring (Gastroesophageal junction/ring)—commonly identified in barium swallow as thin transverse mucosal fold known as B ring.

A ring (Inferior esophageal sphincter) between 2 and 4 cm proximal to B ring, is thicker ring produced by active muscle contraction known as A ring.

Phrenic ampulla (vestibule)—area between these 2 rings A and B, it corresponds with lower esophageal sphincter. It comprises physiologic 2 to 4 cm high pressure zone, which is tightly closed during resting state and assumes bulbous configuration with swallowing.

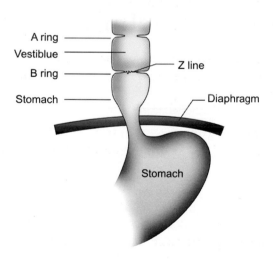

Fig. 1.1: Anatomy of gastroesophageal junction

Z line—the change from squamous epithelium of esophagus to columnar epithelium of stomach in distal esophagus is marked by irregular line called as Z line. Here straight esophageal folds ends abruptly to give rise to gastric rugae.

In case of baretts esophagus (i.e. esophagus lined by columnar epithelium) this line may lie some distance above gastro-esophageal junction. Normally Z line lies at gastro-esophageal junction.

Schatzki Ring

It refers to pathological annular narrowing at B ring, causing dysphagia:

In dysphagia cases ring is   < 12 mm in diameter
In asympotomatic cases ring is   > 20 mm

Common causes are:
- Congenital
- Acquired—due to reflux esophagitis this type is commonly associated with sliding hiatus hernia.

Sliding Hiatal Hernia/Axial Hernia

When esophagogastric junction is >1.5 cm above diaphragmatic hiatus and portion of peritoneal sac forms part of wall of hernia.

Rolling Hiatal Hernia/Paraesophageal Hernia

When portion of stomach is superiorly displaced into thorax and esophagogastric junction remains in subdiaphragmatic position.

ACUTE ESOPHAGITIS

Common radiological findings: These are wide, thickened folds (> 3 mm) with irregular lobulated contour. Vertically oriented ulcers around 3 to 10 mm in length, mucosal erosions and nodularity, inflammatory esophagogastric polyp.

Common causes are:
- Intubation, infection
- Crohn disease, corrosives
- Gastroesophageal reflux/radiation therapy.

ESOPHAGUS

Normal length—25 cm.

Normally—flattened anteroposteriorly, lumen is collapsed. Dilates only during passage of food.

Megaesophagus (Diffuse Esophageal Dilatation)

Common causes are:
- Scleroderma
- Esophagitis
- Idiopathic achalasia
- Benign stricture
- Chagas disease
- Diabetic/alcoholic neuropathy
- Extrinsic compression.

Esophageal Longitudinal Folds

Normally—1 to 2 mm wide, best seen in collapsed esophagus.

Abnormal esophageal folds— > 3 mm wide with submucosal edema/inflammation.

Common causes are:
- Gastroesophageal reflux
- Irradiation
- Opportunistic infection
- Caustic ingestion.

Small Esophageal Ulcer

Size of ulcer is < 1 cm.

Common causes are:
- Reflux esophagitis
- Drug-induced
- Herpes simplex virus type I
- Acute radiation change.

Large Esophageal Ulcer

Size of ulcer is > 1 cm.

Common causes are:
- Carcinoma
- Cytomegalovirus
- Drug-induced
- HIV
- Barrett esophagus.

Focal Esophageal Narrowing

Esophageal stricture—when narrowing is > 10 mm in vertical length.

Esophageal ring—refers to 5 to 10 mm (vertical length) area of complete/incomplete circumferential narrowing.

Esophageal web—refers to 1 to 2 mm thick (vertical length) area of complete/incomplete circumferential narrowing.

Common causes are:
- Tumor
- Esophagitis
- Surgery, scleroderma
- Prolonged nasogastric intubation
- Radiation
- Congenital.

Pneumatosis Cystoides Intestinalis

It refers to presence of multiple 1 to 2 mm gas-filled cysts in wall of stomach and intestine.

Clinically—little or absent gastrointestinal symptoms.

Gastric Pylorus

Normal Measurements
Length   5 to 10 mm
Muscle thickness   Up to 4 mm

Infantile Form of Hypertrophic Pyloric Stenosis

USG findings—pyloric transverse diameter $\geq$ 13 mm with pyloric channel closed elongated pyloric canal $\geq$ 15 mm in length, pyloric muscle wall thickness $\geq$ 4 mm

Pyloric volume >1.4 cc

$3.64 \times$ muscle thickness (mm) + pyloric length > 25 mm

Target sign—hypoechoic ring of hypertrophied pyloric muscle around echogenic mucosa centrally on cross-section.

Benign Gastric Ulcer

Hampton line—refers to thin, straight, 1 mm lucent line, traversing the orifice of the ulcer niche (seen on profile view).

Gastric Volvulus

Based on degrees of rotation, 2 types:

Complete volvulus—when rotation of stomach is > 180°.

Partial volvulus—when rotation of stomach is < 180°, without vascular compromise.

Duodenum

Normal measurements

Length	25 to 30 cm (around 10 inches)
Max width	3 cm

Normal length of different parts

First part	2 inches
Second part	3 inches
Third part	4 inches
Fourth part	1 inch

Dilated Duodenum (> 3 cm Width)

Megabulbus—refers to dilatation of duodenal bulb only.

Megaduodenum—refers to dilatation of entire C-loop

Common causes are:

- Localized ileus, scleroderma, aganglionosis, SLE
- Vascular compression due to abdominal aortic aneurysm, SMA syndrome
- Metastases/inflammatory (pancreatitis, tuberculous enteritis, Crohn's disease).

SUPERIOR MESENTERIC ARTERY SYNDROME/CHRONIC DUODENAL ILEUS

Refers to vascular compression of 3rd part of duodenum within aortomesenteric compartment.

Normal angle between SMA and aorta—45 to 65°

Cause—narrowing of angle to 10 to 22° due to any of the following reasons:

- Asthenic build,
- Weight loss,
- Congenital
- Prolonged bed rest in supine position (surgery, body cast, whole-body burns).

Radiological findings:

Megaduodenum—pronounced dilatation of 1st and 2nd portion of duodenum and frequently stomach abrupt change in caliber distal to compression defect.

Clinically present as—abdominal cramping, repetitive vomiting.

Superior Mesenteric Artery

Normal diameter—< 5 mm.

Origin—1 cm caudal to coeliac axis.

Supplies—transverse and descending duodenum, jejunum, ileum, large bowel to splenic flexure.

Duodenal Ulcer

Commonly < 1 cm, round/ovoid ulcer niche.
Giant duodenal ulcer— > 2 cm.

Jejunal and Ileal Obstruction/Small Bowel Obstruction (SBO)

Measurement findings on **USG:**
- Dilated segment >10 cm in length
- Small bowel loops are dilated, > 3 cm in width

- Collapsed colon
- Increased peristalsis of dilated segment.

Findings in plain abdomen radiograph:
Greater than three distended small bowel loops measuring > 3 cm in diameter with gas-fluid levels (seen > 3–5 hours after onset of obstruction).

Location of obstruction:
Jejunum—when valvulae conniventes high and frequent.

Ileum—when valvulae conniventes sparse/absent.

Common causes are:
- Intrinsic bowel wall inflammation/hemorrhage/ neoplasm/vascular insufficiency
- Jejunal/ileal atresia
- Midgut volvulus, intussusception
- Mesenteric cyst from meconium peritonitis
- Meckel's diverticulum
- Fibrous adhesions from previous surgery
- Luminal occlusion by foreign body/bezoar.

Small Bowel

It is the longest tubular organ in body
Normal length—550 to 600 cm (18–22 feet).

Normal Small Bowel Diameter in Children

Age	Diameter (mm)
1 yr	13.0
5 yr	19.0
10 yr	21.8
15 yr	23.0

Ileocecal Valve

Normal vertical diameter—2.5 cm.
Abnormal—if ≥ 4 cm.

Common abnormalities involved with ileocecal valve are:

- Tuberculosis
- Amebiasis
- Crohn's disease
- Lipomatosis.

Cecal Diameter

Normal range—5-7 cm.
Risk of perforation—if ≥ 9 cm.

Normal Maximum Bowel Caliber

Small bowel	3 cm
Transverse colon	6 cm
Cecum	9 cm

Jejunum

Normal length—10 to 12 feet.

Normal Lumen Diameter

Upper jejunum—3.0 to 4.0 cm
Lower jejunum—2.5 to 3.5 cm
Normal number of folds—4 to 7 inch.
Normal fold thickness—1.7 to 2.0 mm.

Ileum

Normal length	6 to 8 feet
Normal lumen diameter	2.0 to 2.8 cm

| *Normal number of folds* | 2 to 4 inch |
| *Normal fold thickness* | 1.4 to 1.7 mm |

ABNORMAL SMALL BOWEL FOLDS

Jejunum—> 7 folds/inch, > 7 mm fold height , > 2.5 mm fold thickness.

Ileum—> 4 folds/inch, > 3.5 mm fold height, > 2 mm fold thickness.

Common causes are:
- Crohn's disease, infectious enteritis
- Mesenteric lymphadenopathy
- Parasitic infestation/giardiasis
- Malabsorption syndrome
- Zollinger-Ellison syndrome.

TOXIC MEGACOLON

It refers to acute transmural fulminant colitis with neurogenic loss of motor tone and rapid development of extensive colonic dilatation > 5.5 cm involving transverse colon.

Common causes are:
- Ulcerative colitis
- Ischemic colitis
- Pseudomembranous colitis
- Crohn's disease.

APPENDICITIS (FIG. 1.2)

USG measurement findings:
Appendix visualized as noncompressible, blind-ending, tubular aperistaltic structure, laminated wall with target appearance, mural wall thickness $\geq$ 2 mm, $\geq$ 6 mm in total

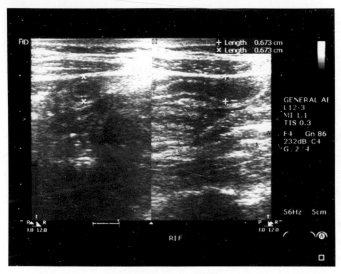

Fig. 1.2: Appendicitis

diameter on cross-section, pericecal/periappendiceal fluid, enlarged mesenteric lymph nodes.

INTUSSUSCEPTION

USG measurement findings:
Target sign—concentric ring of bowel, peripheral rim hypoechogenic 8 mm thick, total diameter on cross-section is > 3 cm.

Ascariasis

It is the most common parasitic infection in world.

Normal measurements:
Length—20 to 30 cm
Width—6 mm

Common location—jejunum > ileum > duodenum
Common age group affected— 1 to 10 years
Life cycle—infection spreads from contaminated soil, eggs hatch in duodenum, larvae penetrate into lymphatics/ venules, then carried to lungs, goes to alveoli, bronchial tree, later swallowed, and matures in jejunum.

On Barium Study

Seen as 20 to 30 cm long tubular filling defects, barium-filled enteric canal is outlined within Ascaris, whirled appearance, sometimes in coiled clusters.
Clinically present as:
- Colic
- Appendicitis
- Hematemesis.

If bile ducts infested—leads to jaundice.

Measurement findings on **USG**—seen as tubular echogenic filling defect with 2 to 4 mm wide central sonolucent line within dilated common bile duct.

Hemoperitoneum Score (HP Score)

This is mainly applied in case of trauma to abdomen, for taking decision for surgical intervention, focused assessment with sonography for trauma (FAST).

HP score = Depth of largest fluid collection in cm + 1 point for each additional site with fluid score of ≤ 2 managed conservatively.

Presacral Space (Fig. 1.3)

It refers to the the shortest distance between the posterior rectum and sacrum.

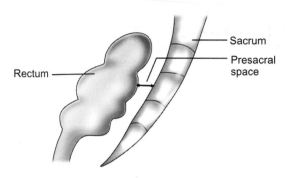

Fig. 1.3: Presacral space

Normal Range

In children	1 to 5 mm
In adults	2 to 16 mm
In older persons	Up to 20 mm

Common causes of enlarged presacral space are:
- *Rectal infection*—proctitis (TB, diverticulitis)
- *Rectal inflammation*—Crohn colitis, ulcerative colitis
- *Sacral tumor*—chordoma, sacrococcygeal teratoma
- Prostatic carcinoma, bladder tumors, cervical cancer, ovarian cancer
- *Rectal tumors*—lipoma, lymphoma, sarcoma, lymph node metastases.
- Collection of pus, hematoma, fat in the presacral space.

Rectosigmoid Index

- Refers to ratio of largest diameter of rectum to the largest diameter of sigmoid colon
- > 1—normal/meconium plug syndrome
- < 1—Hirschsprung disease.

Chapter 2

Genitourinary System

NORMAL KIDNEYS SIZE

In newborn,
Length   4 cm
Width   cm
    <1 yr   4.98 + 0.155 × age (months)
    >1 yr   6.79 + 0.22 × age (year)

RENAL SIZE IN PREMATURE INFANTS

Body weight	Renal length (Range)
600 gm	26.4 to 35.7 mm
1000 gm	29.4 to 38.7 mm
1500 gm	33.4 to 42.5 mm
2000 gm	36.9 to 46.2 mm
2400 gm	39.9 to 49.2 mm

NORMAL RENAL SIZE IN NEWBORN TERM INFANT

	RK (mm)	LK (mm)
Male	41.2 ± 4.4	42.7 ± 4.8
Female	41.8 ± 3.2	42.7 ± 3.7

ADULTS

Length	10-12 cm
Parenchymal width	1.3-2.5 cm
Width	4-6 cm
Respiratory mobility (Craniocaudally)	3-7 cm

RENAL CORTICAL INDEX (RCI) (FIG. 2.1)

Measurements—(in mm)
w- distance between upper and lower poles of kidney

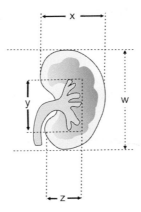

Fig. 2.1: Renal cortical index

x = distance between lateral and medial borders of kidney
y = distance between superior and inferior calyx
z = distance between medial and lateral borders of calyces

Renal cortical index—y × z/w × x

Normal value—0.35 ± 0.04 mm

Significance—it acts as Indicator of functional ability of kidney. In pathological states RCI increases.

ULTRASOUND IN RENAL TRANSPLANT

Normal range
  Cortical thickness (CT)—9.3 -9.7 mm ± 1.5
  Medullary pyramid index (MPI)—½ PL × PW/CT
  Mean value—5.3- 7.0 ± 2.0 cm
  Abnormal range—> 8-9 cm
  PL—pyramid length
  PW—pyramid width

RENAL TRANSPLANT REJECTION FEATURES

- Thinning of cortex and swelling of pyramid
- AP dimension greater than width
- Increased renal size
- Decreased renal sinus fat.

**Normal Ureter Diameter in IVP
(for infants and children)**

Ureteral diameter— 0.187 × age (yrs) + 3.89

Renal Artery

Normal diameter— 6.5 to 6.7 mm

Decreased diameter indicates—reduced renal function

Right renal artery origin—10 clock position

Left renal artery origin—4 clock position

Parenchyma-Pelvis Index (PPI)

Refers to the ratio between the width of the peripheral hypoechoic parenchyma and the width of the central hyperechoic pelvic complex.

In < 30 yrs   > 1.6 : 1
In 30- 60 yrs   1.2- 1.6 : 1
In > 60 yrs   1.1 : 1

Significance of PPI—in chronic renal patients, this ratio increases with age.

ANTERIOR JUNCTION LINE

- Refers to the echogenic line that extends from the renal sinus to the perinephric fat

- Most common location—at the junction of upper and middle third of kidney
- Differential diagnosis—renal scars/angiomyolipoma.

Unilateral Large Smooth Kidney

When measurement > 12 cm in length, > 6 cm in width
Difference of more than 2 cm in length is abnormal

Common causes are
- Acute bacterial nephritis
- Obstructive uropathy
- Crossed fused ectopia
- Adult polycystic kidney
- Multicystic dysplastic kidney
- Acute arterial infarction
- Renal vein thrombosis.

Bilateral Large Kidneys

Common causes are:
- *Bilateral hydronephrosis*—congenital/acquired
- Acute bacterial nephritis
- Acute arterial infarction, renal vein thrombosis
- Leukemia/multiple myeloma/lymphoma/Wilms' tumor
- Polycystic kidney disease
- SLE.

Unilateral Small Kidney (<7 cm in length)

Common causes are:
- Chronic infarction
- Congenital hypoplasia
- Renal artery stenosis
- Radiation nephritis

- Reflux nephropathy
- Postobstructive atrophy

Bilateral Small Kidneys

Common causes are:
- Chronic glomerulonephritis/Papillary necrosis
- Atheroembolic disease/Generalized arteriosclerosis
- Arterial hypotension
- Benign and malignant nephrosclerosis.

Renal Calculi

Radiopaque calculi on USG
When size
> 5 mm–echogenic with distal acoustic shadowing
< 5 mm–echogenic with weak acoustic shadowing.

Ureter

Normal measurements:
Length—30-34 cc
Diameter— < 3 mm

Ureteral Dilatation (> 3 mm Diameter)

Common causes are:
- Chronic vesicoureteral reflux
- Ureterolithiasis
- Megaureter/posterior urethral valves
- Compression by abdominal/pelvic mass.

Megaureter—When size is > 7 mm in diameter
Common causes are:
- Congenital primary megaureter
- Primary reflux megaureter

- Prune belly syndrome
- Secondary vesicoureteral reflux due to posterior urethral valves/neurogenic bladder/bladder outlet obstruction
- Primary obstruction due to ureterocele, stone, tumor, stricture
- Secondary obstruction due to bladder wall mass/ Retroperitoneal tumor/fibrosis.

Renal Pelvis width in Newborn

< 5 mm	normal
5- 10 mm	recquires follow-up
> 10 mm	suspicious for pathologic dilatation.

Multicystic Dysplastic Kidney (Potter Type II)

USG findings are:
Dysplastic kidney so normal renal architecture replaced by—
random cysts of different shape and size (cluster of grapes) with largest cyst in peripheral nonmedial location, usually unilateral.

- Absence of central sinus complex
- Cysts are separated by septa and there is no communication between multiple cysts
- Cysts begin to disappear in infancy
- Corticomedullary differentiation is lost
- Oligohydramnios.

Polycystic Kidney Disease/Adult Polycystic Kidney Disease (Potter Type III)

Clinically,
- Symptomatic at mean age of 35 years
- Abdominal/lumbar pain

- Hypertension
- Proteinuria and hematuria

Ob-USG:
- Large echogenic kidneys similar to infantile PCKD, can be unilateral
- Macroscopic cysts
- Normal amount of amniotic fluid/oligohydramnios.

USG findings are:
- Multiple cysts are present in cortical region, almost always bilateral
- Diffusely echogenic, when size of cysts are small (i.e. during childhood)
- Renal contour is poorly demarcated.

Criteria for screening exam for cyst:

18-29 years   ≥ 5 cysts
30-44 years   ≥ 6 cysts
45-59 years   ≥ 9 in males cysts, ≥ 6 in females

Commonly associated with:
- Cysts in liver, pancreas; rarely in lung, spleen, testis, thyroid, uterus, ovaries
- Mitral valve prolapse
- Saccular berry aneurysm of cerebral arteries/aorta.

Acquired Cystic Kidney Disease

Common in—patients with renal failure undergoing hemodialysis/peritoneal dialysis

USG findings—3-5 cyst of size ranging from 0.5–3 cm, in both cortex and medulla, cyst undergone hemorrhage will give internal echoes.

Adrenal

Normal size (cm)
Neonate

Length	0.9 to 3.6
Thickness	0.2 to 0.5
Width	2 to 2.5

Adult

Length	4 to 6
Thickness	0.2 to 0.6
Width	2 to 3

Each limb of adrenal gland should not be thicker than the crus of the diaphragm.

DIFFERENTIALS OF FOCAL UNILATERAL ADRENAL MASS

Adenocarcinoma—large focal mass (>4 cm) with central necrosis in one adrenal gland and atrophy of contralateral gland.

Adenoma— focal mass (2–4 cm) in one adrenal gland and atrophy of contralateral gland.

Urinary Bladder

Volume of urinary bladder —length × breadth × height × 0.5 postvoid residual volume is significant when > 50 ml

In these cases rule out- bladder outlet obstruction
Normal bladder capacity [in mL] = (age in yrs + 2) × 30

For example,
2 year—up to 120 ml
3 year—up to 150 ml
4 year—up to 180 ml

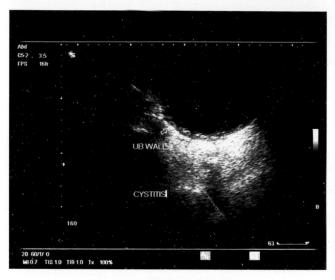

Fig. 2.2: Bladder wall thickening

Normal Capacity

Adult males   <750 ml
Adult females   <550 ml

Bladder Wall Thickening (Fig. 2.2)

Normal bladder wall thickness (irrespective of gender and age)
In well-distended bladder   < 4 mm
In empty bladder   < 8 mm

Common causes of increased thickening
- Cystitis
- Neurogenic bladder
- Tumors
- Bladder outlet obstruction.

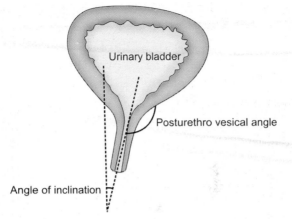

Fig. 2.3: Stress incontinence

Stress Incontinence (Fig. 2.3)

Following angles are calculated on chain cystourethrography.

- *Posterior urethrovesical angle (PUVA)*—it is the angle between posterior aspect of urethra and the base of bladder
  Normal range—90-100 °
- *Angle of inclination of urethra (AI)*—it is the angle formed by extending a line through direction of the upper urethra to join a line in the vertical axis of the patient
  Normal range—10-30 °
  Type I stress in continence—AI > 100°
  Type II stress incontinence—AI > 100° and PUVA > 45°

Testis

Newborn
Normal length   1 to 1.5 cm

Adult

Length	3 to 5 cm
Width	2 to 4 cm
Average transverse diameter	2 cm
Average vertical diameter	2.5 cm
Average size of testis	3.8 × 3.0 × 2.5 cm (decreases with age)

Testicular Microlithiasis

USG findings are—1- 2 mm, hyperechoic, nonshadowing foci (>5) are scattered throughout the parenchyma of both testes distribution may be asymmetrical, unilateral, clustered in periphery.

Associated with—cryptorchidism, granulomas, infertility, testicular germ cell tumor, Klinefelter's syndrome, testicular infarcts.

Epididymis (Fig. 2.4)

It refers to tortuous tightly folded canal forming the efferent route from testis;

It consists of 3 parts—head, body and tail

Normal measurements

Total length	6-7 cm
Head measures	10-12 diameter
body measures	< 4 mm diameter

Note- Epididymal cysts of up to 4 mm diameter commonly occur in 30% of normal individuals.

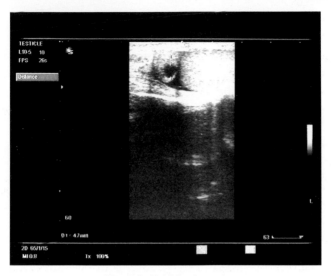

Fig. 2.4: Epididymis cyst

Seminal Vesicle

Normal width in adult	11 ± 2 mm
Seminal vesicle atrophy	When width is < 7 mm
Seminal vesicle hypoplasia	When width is between 7 to 11 mm

Prostate

Normal size

Craniocaudal	< 3 cm
Anteroposterior	< 3 cm
Transverse	< 5 cm

Volume prostate—A × B × C × 0.5
Normal value— < 25 ml

Benign Ductal Ectasia of Prostate
Common in—older age
Findings on USG—1-2 mm diameter tubular structures in peripheral zone of prostate, starts at capsule and radiates towards urethra.

Male Urethra

Normal Length   18 to 20 cm

Female Urethra

Normal measurements
Length   3 to 5 cm
Diameter   6 mm

Scrotal Wall Thickness

Normal value- 2-8 mm
Common causes of scrotal wall thickening (> 8 mm) are:
- Torsion of testis/epididymal or testicular appendage
- Epididymoorchitis
- Trauma
- Acute idiopathic scrotal edema.

Chapter 3

Respiratory System

NORMAL TRACHEA

Age	Length (cm)	AP diameter (cm)
0-2 yr	5.4 ± 0.7	0.53 ±0.10
4-6 yr	7.2 ± 0.8	0.8± 0.06
8-10 yr	8.8± 0.9	1.05±0.05
12-14 yr	10.8± 1.5	1.3 ±0.18
18-20 yr	13.1 ±0.9	1.75± 0.17

Tracheal Bifurcation Level

Newborn	– at	T 3 vertebrae
10-year-old	– at	T 5 vertebrae
Adult	– at	T 6 vertebrae

Widening of Paratracheal Space (> 5 mm)

Normal width is — < 5 mm

Common causes of widening are

- Bronchogenic carcinoma
- Dilated tortuous vessels (SVC, brachiocephalic artery, azygos vein)
- Enlarged lymph node
- Mediastinal hematoma/lipomatosis.

CAVITY

Refers to gas filled space surrounded by complete wall which is ≥ 3 mm:

Common causes are:

- Tuberculosis
- Pneumoconiosis
- Malignancy
- Abscess

- Bulles, blebs
- Bronchogenic cyst/traumatic lung cyst.

Coarse Reticulations

Following are the radiological features
- Honeycomb lung
- Rounded radiolucencies <1 cm in areas of increased lung density
- Coarse reticular interstitial densities with intervening cystic spaces
- Decreased lung volume.

Commonly seen in
- *Granulomatous disease*—sarcoidosis, eosinophilic granuloma.
- Pneumoconioses.
- Drug hypersensitivity, radiotherapy.
- *Collagen-vascular disease*—scleroderma, rheumatoid lung.

Nodular Lung Disease

Macronodular Lung Disease

Refers to nodules >5 mm in diameter
Commonly seen in
- Abscess, AVM, Amyloidosis
- Granuloma (fungus, eosinophilic granuloma)
- Multiple myeloma, metastases
- *Echinococcus.*

Micronodular Lung Disease

Refers to discrete 3 to 5 mm small, round, focal opacity commonly seen in:

- Pneumoconiosis
- Histiocytosis X
- Granulomatous disease (miliary TB, histoplasmosis)
- Chickenpox.

Bronchiole

- Normal bronchiole— < 1 mm
- Dilated bronchiole— > 2 mm.

Pulmonary Nodule/Mass

Refers to pulmonary or pleural-based, sharply defined, discrete, nearly circular opacity

Mass—When size is > 30 mm in diameter

Nodule—When size is 2 to 30 mm in diameter

Common causes are–

- *Malignant tumors*—Metastases/Bronchogenic carcinoma/ lymphoma/sarcoma
- *Benign tumors*—AVM, lipoma, Bronchogenic cyst, hamartoma, fibroma
- *Infections*—Round pneumonia/Rounded atelectasis, tuberculosis, histoplasmosis, abscess, hydatid cyst, bronchiectatic cyst, bronchocele.

Morphologic Evaluation of Solitary Pulmonary Nodule

- Cavitation
  - A thick irregular wall (>16 mm) is suggestive of malignant nodule
  - A thin smooth wall ($\leq$ 4 mm) is benign in 94 percent.
- Size
  - Smaller the nodule the more likely it is benign

- When nodule < 20 mm — in 80 percent of cases it is benign
- When nodule > 30 mm — in > 93 percent of cases it is malignant.

Note: Pulmonary nodule evaluation needs further correlation with other findings like — margins, calcification, satellite lesion, contrast enhancement and doubling time.

Acquired Cyst

Bulla—it refers to sharply demarcated dilated airspace within lung parenchyma >1 cm in diameter with <1 mm wall thickness, due to destruction of alveoli.

Bleb—it refers to cystic air collection within visceral pleura; mostly apical with narrow neck; commonly associated with spontaneous pneumothorax.

Pneumothorax Size (Fig. 3.1)

Average interpleural distance (in cm) = $(P + Q + R) \div 3$

Diaphragm

Normal thickness— 5 mm
Covered by
- Parietal pleura on thoracic side
- Peritoneum on abdomen side.

Azygos Vein

On erect chest radiograph, normal diameter of azygos vein- ≤ 7 mm

Common causes of dilatation of azygos vein are:
- SVC or IVC obstruction/compression
- Portal hypertension

- Pregnancy
- Hepatic vein occlusion
- Large pericardial effusion
- Right-sided heart failure.

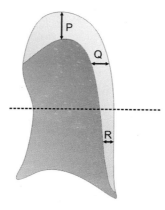

Fig. 3.1: PA view left lung

P Refers to maximum apical interpleural distance
Q Refers to interpleural distance at midpoint of upper half of lung
R Refers to interpleural distance at midpoint of lower half of lung

Scale for Measurement of Pneumothorax

Avg Interpleural distance (cm)	% Pneumothorax	
	Supine	Erect
0.5	14%	9%
1.0	19%	14%
2.0	29%	22.5%
3.0	39%	31.5%
4.0	49%	40%
5.0	59%	49%

Normal Position of Tracheal Tube

Ideal location is when tip of tube—4 to 6 cm above carina with neck in neutral position:
- Migration by 2 cm inferiorly with flexion
- Migration by 2 cm superiorly with extension
- *Tube diameter*—should be 1/2 to 2/3 of tracheal lumen
- Diameter of inflated balloon should be less than diameter of trachea.

Tracheostomy Tube

Ideal site for tip is 1/2 to 2/3rd the distance from the stoma to the carina.

NG Tube

Side holes in NG tube extend from tip till 10 cm of length, so ideally last 10 cm of tube should be in stomach.

Pulmonary Artery Catheter

Ideal location for swan ganz catheter tip is within 2 cm of pulmonary hilum on a frontal radiograph.

Pleural Drain Tube

- *For draining fluid*—Tube should be placed at level of 6 to 8th, intercostal space, postero inferiorly in mid axillary line.
- *For air drainage*—Tube should be placed at the level of 2nd intercostal space, antero superiorly in anterior axillary line.

EMPHYSEMA

Refers to group of pulmonary diseases having permanently enlarged air spaces distal to terminal bronchioles accompanied by destruction of alveolar walls.

Chest Radiograph Findings

- Hyperinflated lung, bullae
- Retrosternal air space >2.5 cm
- Barrel chest– refers to enlarged A-P chest diameter
- Flat hemidiaphragm (distance between line connecting the cardio- and costophrenic angles and top of mid hemidiaphragm <1.5 cm)
- Low hemidiaphragm
- Pulmonary vascular pruning and distortion.

Chronic Pulmonary Thromboembolism

Radiological measurement findings on CT
- Pulmonary hypertension
- Right and left pulmonary arteries > 18 mm in diameter
- Main pulmonary artery diameter > 28.6 mm
- Cardiomegaly
- Hypertrophy of right atrium and right ventricle
- Transverse diameter of RV > 45 mm
- Transverse diameter of RA > 35 mm.

TRACHEOBRONCHOMEGALY

Refers to primary dysplasia/atrophy of supporting structures of trachea and major bronchi with abrupt transition to normal bronchi at 4th to 5th division.

Radiological Measurement Findings

Marked dilatation of
- Trachea (> 29 mm)
- Left mainstem bronchi (>15 mm)
- Right mainstem bronchi (> 20 mm).

TRACHEAL INDEX

Refers to the ratio of coronal and sagittal diameters to trachea.

Normal Values

- In men— < 1
- In women and children—close to 1.

Significance

For example, In COPD patients (sabre sheath trachea) tracheal index is less than 0.6.

Chapter 4

Cardiovascular System

HEART VALVE POSITIONS ON CHEST RADIOGRAPH

PA View

Reference line–it refers to oblique line drawn from distal left mainstem bronchus to right cardiophrenic angle

- Mitral valve is situated inferior to this line, centrally located within cardiac silhouette
- Pulmonary valve is situated just inferior to left mainstem bronchus
- Tricuspid valve inferior to this line more basilar and midline
- Aortic valve is situated superior to this line, overlying the thoracic spine

Main Pulmonary Artery

Normal diameter (adult)–22 ± 3 mm

Decreased Diameter of Pulmonary Artery

Commonly seen in:
- Chronic thromboembolic disease
- Lung cancer
- Mediastinal fibrosis.

Dilatation of Pumonary Artery

Commonly seen in:

- Pulmonary arterial hypertension
- Pulmonary valve stenosis
- Aneurysm
- Pulmonary regurgitation.

Pulmonary Hypertension

Common causes are:
- Chronic thromboembolic disease
- Connective tissue disorder—CREST, Scleroderma
- Pulmonary vasculitis,
- COPD
- Left to right shunt.

Radiological measurement findings on CT

Vascular Signs
- Main pulmonary artery diameter >29 mm
- Diameter of left and right pulmonary artery >16 mm
- Segmental artery-to-bronchus ratio >1 in three lobes
- Ratio of main pulmonary artery diameter to aorta diameter ratio >1
- Enlarged bronchial systemic arteries >1.5 mm
- Pruning of peripheral pulmonary arteries
- Enlarged pulmonary veins secondary to left-sided heart disease
- Small pulmonary veins secondary to precapillary pulmonary HTN.

Mediastinal and Cardiac Signs
- RV myocardial thickness >4 mm
- Right heart dilatation, i.e. ratio of RV:LV> 1:1
- Dilatation of IVC and coronary sinus
- Mild pericardial thickening/small pleural effusion.

Inferior Vena Cava

Origin—formed by paired common iliac vein at anterior surface of L 5 vertebrae

Entry to right atrium—at the level of T8 vertebrae
- Normal diameter in adult   < 20 mm
- Normal diameter in young athletes   < 25 mm

Variation in diameter with respiration:

On deep inspiration—diameter increases, because of decrease venous return

On deep expiration—diameter decreases, because of increase venous return

Right Atrial Enlargement

PA view chest radiograph findings:
- Most lateral RA margin >2.5 cm from right vertebral margin and >5.5 cm from midline
- Prominent round superior border at junction with SVC.

Common causes are:
- Atrial septal defect
- Tricuspid stenosis/regurgitation,
- Pulmonary atresia
- Ebstein anomaly.

Right Heart Failure

*Common **USG** findings are:*
- IVC is dilated — > 20 mm/>25 mm in young athletes
- Hepatic veins are dilated (at periphery) — > 6 mm
- IVC is not collapsed during forced inspiration
- Pleural effusion.

Left Atrial Enlargement

PA view chest radiograph findings—
- >75° splaying of carina and horizontal orientation of distal left mainstem bronchus

- Distance between midpoint of undersurface of left mainstem bronchus and right lateral LA shadow measures > 7.5 cm (male)/7.0 (female)
- Right retrocardiac double density
- Enlarged left-convex left atrial appendage ± calcifications.

Common causes are:
- Congenital   – PDA, VSD
- Acquired   – LV failure, mitral regurgitation/stenosis, LA myxoma

Pericardial Effusion (Fig. 4.1)

Criteria—When pericardial fluid is >50 ml

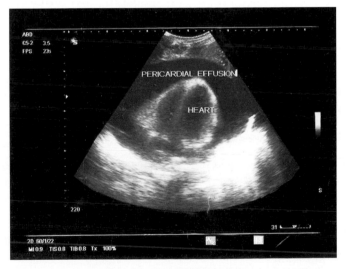

Fig. 4.1: Pericardial effusion

Chest Radiograph Findings

- *Water bottle configuration*— symmetrically enlarged cardiac silhouette
- Loss of retrosternal clear space
- Normal radiograph when fluid is <250 ml/in acute pericarditis
- *Fat-pad sign*—separation of retrosternal from epicardial fat line >2 mm by water density
- *Clinically present*—with fatigue, dyspnea and symptoms of cardiac tamponade.

Common causes are:

- Congestive heart failure, myxedema
- Penetrating/nonpenetrating trauma
- Cardiac surgery/catheterization, chemotherapy, radiation
- Acute myocardial infarction/rupture
- Rupture of ascending aorta/pulmonary trunk.

Pericardium

Normal pericardial thickness–1 to 3 mm

Constrictive Pericarditis

It refers to fibrous thickening of pericardium which interferes with filling of ventricular chambers through restriction of heart motion.

CT Findings

- Epicardium >2 mm thick
- Dilatation of SVC and IVC
- *Common age group*—30 to 50 year

- *Common causes are:*
  - Tuberculosis
  - Cardiac surgery trauma
  - Radiotherapy to mediastinum
  - Idiopathic
  - Chronic renal failure

AORTOVERTEBRAL DISTANCE

- It refers to the distance between posterior aortic wall and the anterior vertebral borders
  Normally— < 5 mm
- In case of retroaortic space occupying lesion—distance > 5 mm.

Thoracic Aortic Aneurysm

Normal average diameter of thoracic aorta
- Aortic root   – 3.6 cm
- Ascending aorta 1 cm proximal to arch   – 3.5 cm
- Arch   – 2.9 cm
- Proximal descending aorta   – 2.6 cm
- Middle descending aorta   – 2.5 cm
- Distal descending aorta   – 2.4 cm

- *Arteriomegaly*— generalized enlargement of arteries
- *Aortic aneurysm* — when diameter is >5 cm
- *Aortic ectasia* — when diameter is 4-5 cm
- *Risk for rupture* — when diameter is >10 cm
- *Common cause* is atherosclerosis.

Clinically present as:
- SVC syndrome (due to venous compression)
- Substernal/back/shoulder pain

- Dysphagia (due to esophageal compression)
- Hoarseness (due to recurrent laryngeal nerve compression)
- Stridor, dyspnea (due to tracheobronchial compression).

Normal Size of Adult Abdominal Aorta

Upper 1/3	– 2 to 3 cm
Middle 1/3	– 1.5 to 2.5 cm
Lower 1/3	– 1 to 2 cm
Aortic ectasia	– 2.5 to 3 cm
Aneurysm	– > 3 cm

Normal Size of Right and Left Common Iliac Arteries

Females	<12 mm
Males	< 14 to 15 mm

Right and Left Common Femoral Arteries – *< 11 mm*

Enlarged Aorta

Common causes

- Aortic coarctation
- Aortic valvular stenosis
- Systemic hypertension
- Syphilitic aortitis
- Traumatic/atherosclerotic aneurysm
- PDA.

PA view chest radiograph findings:
- Aortic knob distance measured from indented trachea to most lateral margin of aorta is >4.0 cm
- Right convex contour above RA margin and lateral displacement of SVC.

Abdominal Aortic Aneurysm (AAA)

It refers to focal widening of aorta >3 cm

Increased risk for rupture when
- Growth is >5 mm every 6 months
- If size >6 cm
- Diverticular rather than fusiform
- E/o dissection.

Clinically present with—sudden severe abdominal pain ± radiating into back, faintness, syncope, hypotension

Surgery recommended—if >5 cm in diameter.

Chapter 5

Central Nervous System

PINEAL GLAND

Function— regulates short and long term biological rhythm

Normal measurements:

Length – 8 mm

Width – 4 mm

Physiological Pineal calcification—common in 2/3 of adult population

Appearance—amorphous/ringlike calcification

Situation and size—< 3 mm from midline and usually <10 mm in diameter

Note: Pineal calcification >14 mm suggests pineal neoplasm (teratoma/pinealoma)

Pineal Gland Localization (Fig. 5.1)

Radiograph—lateral skull

Note: This method is used when pineal gland is visible as a result of calcification

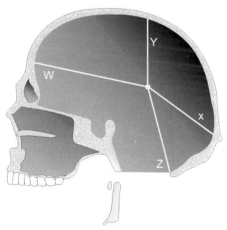

Fig. 5.1: Skull—lateral radiograph

Important landmarks are:

W—Refers to greatest distance from the pineal gland to the inner table of the frontal bone

X—Refers to greatest distance from the pineal gland to the inner aspect of the occipital bone

Y—Refers to greatest distance from the pineal gland to the table of the skull vertex

Z—Refers to greatest distance from the pineal gland to the posterior margin of the foramen magnum.

Significance

Pineal shift may be caused by—tumor, hemorrhage or localized atrophic disease

Measurement W and X—used for assessing anterior or posterior displacement

Measurement Y and Z—used for assessing superior or inferior displacement.

Normal Values of CSF Spaces in Newborn

Sinocortical width	< 3 mm
Craniocortical width	< 4 mm
Interhemispheric width	< 6 mm
Width of 3rd ventricle	< 10 mm
Width of lateral ventricle, frontal horn	< 13 mm

Ventriculomegaly

Common Causes

- Hydrocephalus
- Neoplasm
- TORCH

- Alcohol, drugs, toxins
- Holoprosencephaly
- Porencephaly/Hydranencephaly/Schizencephaly

Ventricle Size Index

This is used to assess the size of the ventricles calculated by taking the ratio of width of the ventricle to width of a hemisphere at widest part of the skull.

Normal value— < 0.33

Ventriculomegaly— >0.33

HYDROCEPHALUS

It refers to excess of CSF due to imbalance of CSF formation and absorption which results in increased intraventricular pressure.

Congenital Hydrocephalus

Ob-USG *measurement findings-*
- Lateral width of ventricular atrium ≥10 mm
- BPD >95th percentile
- Polyhydramnios

Dangling choroid plexus sign—Downside choroid plexus falling away from medial wall and hanging from tela choroidea and upside choroid falling away from lateral wall.

Skull Radiograph Findings (in Newborn/Infant)

- Increase in craniofacial ratio
- Bulging of anterior fontanel
- Sutural diastasis
- Macrocephaly and frontal bossing

CT Scan Findings

- Signs favoring hydrocephalus over white matter atrophy
- Commensurate dilatation of temporal horn with lateral ventricles (most reliable sign)
- Dilatation of ventricular system disproportionate to dilatation of cortical sulci
- Mickey Mouse ears on axial scans, rounding of frontal horn shape with enlargement of frontal horn radius
- Narrowing of ventricular angle.

Brainstem

Normal AP Diameter (mm)

Age	Midbrain	Pons	Medulla
2-3 yr	14-17	17-21	8-13
4-5 yr	15-18	18-22	10-13
8-10 yr	16-19	18-24	11-14
16-20 yr	16-19	20-25	11-14
21-50 yr	16-19	21-25	11-14
51-65 yr	15-18	21-25	10-14

Pituitary Gland

Normal size
- Height in adult females   range 4 to 10 mm
- Height in adult males   range 3 to 7 mm

Shape
- Flat/downwardly convex superior border
- Upwardly convex during puberty, pregnancy and hypothyroidism (due to hyperplasia)
  Macroadenoma—>10 mm in size
  Microadenoma—<10 mm in size

Sella Turcica Size

Radiograph—lateral skull

Important Landmarks

AP diameter—It is the widest distance between anterior and posterior surfaces of pituitary fossa normal range is 5 to 16 mm

Vertical diameter—It is distance between fossa floor and the plane between the opposing surfaces of the anterior and posterior clinoid process. Normal range is 4 to 12 mm

Significance

Enlarged sella

Common Causes

- Extra pituitary mass
- Pituitary tumors
- Empty sella syndrome
- A normal variant

Sutural Diastasis

Common Causes

- Hydrocephalus
- Hypoparathyroidism; hypothyroidism
- Hypo/hypervitaminosis A
- Osteogenesis imperfecta, rickets
- Cleidocranial dysplasia
- Intracerebral tumor

Common location—Coronal >sagittal > lambdoid

Criteria for wide sutures

When intersutural distance is

>10 mm at birth,

>3 mm at 2 yrs,

>2 mm at 3 yrs

Note: Sutures are splittable up to 12-15 yrs; and complete closure occurs by 30 year.

**Craniometry of Craniovertebral Junction
(Figs 5.2 and 5.3)**

On lateral view radiograph of skull, following lines and angles are used in craniometry.

Craniovertebral angle (Clivus-canal angle)—It is the angle formed by line drawn along posterior surface of axis body and odontoid process and basilar line [line along clivus]

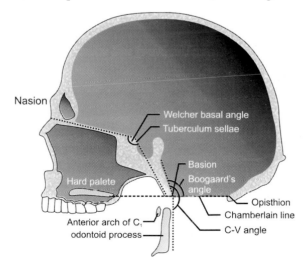

Nasion

Welcher basal angle
Tuberculum sellae

Basion

Boogaard's angle

Hard palate

Opisthion

Chamberlain line

C-V angle

Anterior arch of C₁

odontoid process

Fig. 5.2: Skull lateral view

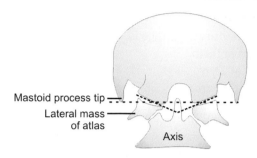

Mastoid process tip

Lateral mass of atlas

Axis

Fig. 5.3: Skull AP view (Open mouth view)

Normally—It ranges from 150° in flexion to 180° in extension

Significance—Angle is decreased, i.e < 150°, in atlanto-occipital assimilation (basilar invagination), platybasia

Welcher Basal Angle

It is the angle formed by tuberculum-basion line and nasion-tuberculum line

Normally—Angle meas <140°

Significance—It is increased, i.e > 140° in platybasia

Chamberlain Line

It is the line between opisthion (posterior margin of foramen magnum) and posterior pole of hard palate

Normally—Tip of odontoid process lies below Chamberlain line

Significance—This line is violated in basilar invagination (condylar/basi occiput hypoplasia), basilar impression

McRae Line

It is the line between posterior lip (opisthion) to anterior lip (basion) of foramen magnum.

Normally—Tip of odontoid lies below this line.

Significance this line is violated in—Basilar invagination, basilar impression.

Boogaard's Angle

It refers to the angle formed by line drawn between basion and the opisthion and line drawn from the dorsum sellae to the basion along the plane of clivus.

Normal range is
   Minimum—119°
   Maximum--135°.

Significance—In basilar impression angle is > 135°

Boogaard's line—It refers to the line connecting the nasion to the opisthion

Normally—Basion should lie below this line.

Significance—In basilar impression, basion will be above Boogaard's line.

On AP View Radiograph of Skull

Bimastoid line–It is the line connecting tips of both mastoid processes
Normally—Tip of odontoid lies <10 mm above this line
Significance—In basilar invagination, (condylar hypoplasia) tip of odontoid lies >10 mm above this line.

Atlanto-occipital joint axis angle
It is the angle formed by lines drawn parallel to both atlanto-occipital joints

These lines intersect at center of odontoid process.

Normal range is—24° to 127°

Significance–Angle is widened in basilar invagination

Few Other Important Lines

George's Line (Posterior Vertebral Alignment Line)

Radiograph—Lateral cervical spine

Important landmarks—Posterior vertebral body surfaces are connected with a continuous line that traverses the intervertebral disk. Also note that a straight line cannot be drawn because of the normal concavity of superior and inferior posterior body corners.

Significance

If retro or anterolisthesis is present, this may be a radiologic sign of instability caused by, dislocation, fracture, ligamentous laxity, or degenerative joint disease.

Posterior Cervical Line (Spinolaminar Junction Line)

Radiograph—Lateral cervical spine radiograph (flexion, neutral, extension)

Important landmarks—Spinolaminar junction is first identified at each level C1 to C7. Each spinolaminar junction will be curved slightly anteriorly from superior to inferior.

Normal measurement—On joining each spinolaminar junction point, a smooth arc- like curve is formed, also at the C2 level, the spinolaminar junction line in children should not exceed 2 mm anterior to this line.

Significance

- A disruption in the line, may be a sign of retro or anterolisthesis, or frank dislocation
- It is especially useful for detection of atlantoaxial subluxation (anterior) and subtle odontoid fractures.

Some More Normal Dimensions in Adults

- Atlanto-occipital articulation   < 2 mm
- Anterior atlanto-dens interval   < 2 mm
- Atlantoaxial articulation   < 3 mm
- Lateral atlanto-dens interval   < 3 mm
- Prevertebral soft tissues at C2   < 6 mm

Normal Values for Cervical Prevertebral Soft Tissues

Level	Neutral (mm)	Flexion (mm)	Extension (mm)
C1	10	11	8
C2	5	6	6
C3	7	7	6
C4	7	7	8
C5	20	22	20
C6	20	20	19
C7	20	20	21

Note:

- In patients > 82 kg—add 1 mm to these normal range.
- In patients > 70 yrs—values may be 1 mm less than normal range.

Atlantoaxial Subluxation

It refers to displacement of atlas with respect to axis.

Types—anterior/posterior

Few common causes are:
- Morquio/Down/Marfan syndrome
- Occipitalization of atlas
- Aplasia of dens
- Rheumatoid/psoriatic arthritis
- Retropharyngeal abscess, otitis media, cervical adenitis, mastoiditis.

Anterior atlantoaxial subluxation
Measurement findings are:
- Retrodental space— < 18 mm
- Predental space— > 2.5 mm; > 4.5 mm (in children)

Atlanto-occipital Dislocation

Common cause—Rapid deceleration with hyperflexion or hyperextension

Clinically—Symptoms range from respiratory arrest with quadriplegia to normal neurologic examination

Direction of dislocation/subluxation can be—Posteriorly, anteriorly, or superiorly

Lateral Radiograph Measurement Findings

Anterior subluxation findings (Fig. 5.4)
- Basion-dens interval (BD) >12 mm
- Powers ratio—BC/OA >1
- It is the ratio of distance between basion and spinolaminar line of C1 (C) and the distance between posterior cortex of anterior tubercle of C1 and opisthion
- >10 mm soft-tissue swelling anterior to C2

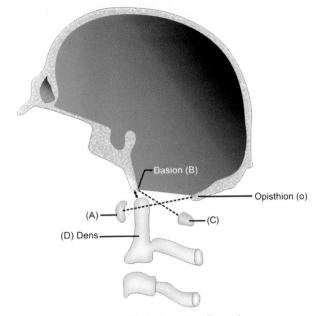

Fig. 5.4: Skull—lateral radiograph

- Basion-axial interval >12 mm anterior to posterior axial line
- Basion-axial interval > 4 mm posterior to posterior axial line.

Sagittal Dimension of the Cervical Spinal Canal

Radiograph—Lateral cervical spine (flexion, neutral, extension)

Important landmarks—Sagittal diameter is measured from the posterior surface of the midvertebral body to the same segmental spinolaminar junction line.

Normal Range in Adults

Level

C1	-	16 to 31 mm
C2	-	14 to 27 mm
C3	-	13 to 23 mm
C4	-	12 to 22 mm
C5	-	12 to 22 mm
C6	-	12 to 22 mm
C7	-	12 to 22 mm

Significance

When it measures <12 mm—Spinal stenosis

Pavlov's Ratio (Canal to Body Ratio)

Most accurate procedure, ratio of the sagittal dimension of the canal and vertebral body, ratio of less than 0.82 is indicates- spinal stenosis.

Cervical Lordosis

Radiograph—Lateral cervical spine.

Important Landmarks

Angle of cervical curve—Two lines are drawn, one through the mid points of the anterior and posterior tubercles of the atlas (atlas plane line) other through and parallel to the inferior endplate of the C 7 body. Perpendiculars are then constructed to the point of intersection; the resultant angle is measured.

Normal range for cervical lordosis - 35 to 45°

Significance

Reduced curve seen in
- Trauma
- Muscle spasm
- Degenerative spondylosis.

Measurement of Thoracic Scoliosis (Cobb's Method)

Radiograph—AP thoracic spine

End vertebrae—These are 2, each located at the superior and inferior extremes of the scoliosis. These appear as the last segment at the extreme ends of the scoliosis, where the endplates tilt to the side of the curvature concavity.

Endplates lines—these are the lines drawn parallel to respective end plate of superior and inferior end vertebra.

Perpendicular lines—Perpendicular lines to these end plate lines are then constructed and the resultant angle is measured at the intersection of the lines.

Significance

- Scoliosis <20° require no bracing or surgical intervention
- Scoliosis <20°, if present in 10-15 year of age, careful monitoring for progression of 5° or more in any 3 – month period.
- If 20-40°, bracing to prevent progression in the growth period.
- If > 40°, surgical intervention.

Measurement of Thoracic Kyphosis

Radiograph—Lateral thoracic spine

Important landmarks—Line is drawn parallel to through the superior endplate of the T1 body and through the inferior endplate of the T12 body. At right angles to both endplate lines, lines are drawn to intersect, and their resultant angle is measured.

Normal values (in degrees)

Age (Yrs)	Males Range	SD	Females Range	SD
2-9	5-40	8	8-36	7
10-19	8-39	8	11-41	7
20-29	13-48	8	7-40	8
30-39	13-49	8	10-42	9
40-49	17-44	7	21-50	7
50-59	25-45	6	22-53	10
60-69	25-62	5	34-54	8
70-79	32-66	8	30-56	9

Increased kyphosis commonly seen in
- Osteoporosis
- Old age
- Scheuermann's disease
- Muscular paralysis

Lumbar Intervertebral Disk Angles (Fig. 5.5)

Radiograph—Lateral lumbar spine

Important landmarks—Lines are drawn through and parallel to each lumbar body endplate; these are then extended posteriorly until they intersect. The angle formed is then measured.

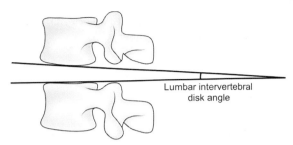

Fig. 5.5: Lumbar spine lateral view

Normal Values for Lumbar Intervertebral Disk Angles

Disk level	Average angle (°)
L1	8
L2	10
L3	12
L4	14
L5	14

Importance

Angle is increased in—In facet syndrome
Angle is reduced in—In acute diskal injuries

Intervertebral Disk Height of Lumbar Spine

Radiograph—Lateral lumbar spine.

Important Landmark

Hurxthal's method—in this method distance between the opposing endplates at the midpoint between the anterior and the posterior vertebral body margins is measured.

Note: When lateral flexion is > 20° or segmental rotation is > 40°, this method is not valid.

Decreased Disk Height

Common Causes

- Infection
- Disk degeneration
- Postsurgery
- Congenital hypoplasia.

Lumbar Spinal Stenosis

Radiological Measurement Findings on MRI

On sagittal view—thecal sac appears in hourglass configuration

On axial view—thecal sac appears as triangular shape sagittal diameter of spinal canal <16 mm (normal range in adults-15-23 mm)

- Dural sac area <100 mm^2
- Bulging disks
- Diminished amount of CSF and crowding of nerve roots thickened articular process, pedicles, laminae, ligaments.

Common Causes

- Spondylolisthesis/achondroplasia/Paget's disease
- Herniated disk
- Metastasis to vertebrae
- Developmental/congenital.

Common age group—30-50 yrs

Clinically—Often asymptomatic until middle age

Low back pain, both lower limbs pain, numbness, weakness worse during walking/standing paraparesis, incontinence (cauda equina syndrome)

Interpediculate Distance

Spinal level	Normal range in adults (mm)
C3	25-31
C4	26-32
C5	26-33
C6	26-33
C7	24-32
T1	20-28
T2	17-24
T3	16-22
T4	15-21
T5	14-21
T6	14-20
T7	14-20
T8	15-21
T9	15-21
T10	15-22
T11	18-24
T12	19-27
L1	21-29
L2	21-30
L3	21-31
L4	21-33
L5	23-36

Sagittal Canal Measurement (Eisenstein's Method) (Fig. 5.6)

Radiograph—Lateral lumbar spine.

Important landmarks—the sagittal canal diameter can be determined by:

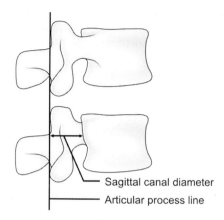

Sagittal canal diameter
Articular process line

Fig. 5.6

Posterior body margin—refers to the measurement point on the posterior body margin which is at the midpoint between the superior and the inferior endplate.

Articular process line—refers to the line connecting the tips of the superior and inferior articular processes at each level.

Sagittal canal measurement—For L1-L4 vertebrae, it is obtained by measuring the distance between the articular process line and the posterior body margin for L5 segment-measurement is made between the spinolaminar junction line and the posterior body.

Significance

If measurement is < 15 mm, at any level, it indicates spinal stenosis.

Wedge-shaped Vertebrae

Commonly seen in—osteoporosis

Measurement findings—anterior border height reduced by >4 mm compared to posterior border height.

Disk Bulge

It refers to the concentric smooth expansion of disk, involving >50% of disk circumference, beyond the confines of endplates.

Herniation of Nucleus Pulposus

It refers to protrusion of disk material >3 mm beyond margins of adjacent vertebral endplates, involving <50% of disk circumference.

Focal Disk Protusion

- It refers to triangular shape of herniation with a base wider than the radius of its depth.
- It involves <25% of disk circumference.

Broad-Based Disk Protrusion

It involves 25–50% of disk circumference.

Disk Extrusion

It refers to mushroom-shaped herniation of disk with base narrower than the radius of its depth (toothpaste sign).

Disk Sequestration (Free Fragment Herniation)

- It refers to complete separation of disk material from parent disk with rupture through posterior longitudinal ligament into epidural space.
- Disk material is noted >9 mm away from intervertebral disk space.

- These migrate superiorly/inferiorly away from disk space with compression of nerve root above/below level of disk herniation.

Normal Location of Tip of Conus Medullaris

16 weeks of gestation	L 4/L 5
Birth	L 2/L 3
>3 months of age	L1- L2

Cord Tethering/Low Conus Medullaris/Tight Filum Terminale Syndrome

It refers to abnormally thick and short filum terminale with position of conus medullaris below L2- L3 at birth.

Tethered Cord

- Conus medullaris is below the level of L3 at birth and below L2 by age 12.
- Abnormal lateral course of nerve roots (>15° relative to spinal cord).
- Widened triangular thecal sac tented posteriorly.

Tight Filum

- Diameter of filum terminale >2 mm at L5 - S1 level
- Small fibrolipoma within thickened filum/small filar cyst.

Vertebrae—lumbar spina bifida occulta with interpedicular widening.

Transforaminal Herniation

It refers to herniation of inferior mesial portions of cerebellum downward through foramen magnum plane-on sagittal/coronal images.

- In children—cerebellar tonsils $\geq$ 7 mm below foramen magnum.
- In adults—cerebellar tonsils $\geq$ 5 mm below foramen magnum.
  For example, chiari-I malformation.

Intracranial Giant Aneurysm

Refers to aneurysm larger than 2.5 cm in diameter, usually presenting with intracranial mass effect

Lacunar Infarction

It refers to small deep infarcts in the distribution of penetrating vessels (lenticulostriate, thalamoperforating and pontine perforating arteries)

Common age group—usually >55 yrs

Risk factors—diabetes/hypertension

Plain CT findings—small hypodense foci measure between 3-15 mm in size (usually <10 mm in diameter)

Microcephaly

Radiological Measurement Findings

- Head circumference <3 SD below the mean
- AC: HC discrepancy
- Ape like sloping of forehead
- Dilatation of lateral ventricles
- *Common causes are*—intrauterine infection-TORCH, drugs, hypoxia, irradiation
- Chromosomal abnormalities (trisomies 13, 18, 21)
  Premature craniosynostosis.

Macrocephaly

Size > 95th percentile

Common Causes

- Hydrocephalus
- Neoplasm.

Choroid Plexus Hemorrhage

Commonly seen in—full-term infants

Common causes are—asphyxia, birth trauma, seizures, apnea

Radiological Measurement Findings

- Enlargement of choroid plexus >12 mm in AP diameter
- Left-right choroids plexus asymmetry >5 mm
- Echogenicity of choroid plexus same as hemorrhage.

Chapter 6

ENT—Orbit

RETROPHARYNGEAL SPACE

It refers to potential space situated behind pharynx.

Normal value
Infants—<3/4 of AP diameter of adjacent cervical spine
Older children—<3 mm

Common causes of retropharyngeal space narrowing are:
- Retropharyngeal abscess
- Hematoma
- Hemangioma
- Branchial cleft cyst
- Cystic hygroma
- Neurofibromatosis.

MAXILLARY SINUS

Visualization by- 2-3 months
Normal values (mm)

	AP diameter	*Width*	*Vertical height*
1yr	14-16	5-6	6-6.5
6yr	27- 28	16-17	16-17
10 yr	30-31	19-20	17.5- 18
18yr	31-33	19-21	20-21

Maxillary Hypoplasia

Common Causes

- Down's syndrome
- Drugs (alcohol, dilantin, valproate)
- Apert/Crouzon syndrome

- Achondroplasia
- Cleft lip/palate

Frontal Sinus

Visualization by–8-10 yr
Normal size (mm) is-

Age	Height	Length	Width
1-2 yr	5	4.5	2.5
7-8 yr	13	8.5	10
10-11 yr	16	9	10
19-20 yr	26	17	26

Sphenoid Sinus

Visualization by-1-2 yr
Normal size (mm)

Age (yr)	Height	Length	Width
1	2.5	1.5	2.5
2	4	2.2	3.5
14	15	7	14

Thyroid Gland

Normal size:
Adult–
Transverse (width)   - 1-2.5 cm
Length (Craniocaudal)   - 3-5 cm
Sagittal   - 1-2.5 cm
Volume of thyroid gland – A × B × C × 0.5
Normal Volume

	Male	*Female*
Newborn	< 3.5	<2.3
1-4 yr	< 3.8	< 4.7
5-10 yr	< 6.0	< 6.5
11-12 yr	< 13.9	< 14.6
Adults	< 25.0	< 18.0

Psammoma Bodies

It refers to microcalcifications Measuring <1 mm and occures in 54% of thyroid neoplasms
Commonly seen in
- Follicular carcinoma
- Papillary carcinoma.

Parathyroid Glands

Total no – 4, two superior and two inferior
Normal Size: 5 × 3 × 1 mm.

Normal Thymus Gland

Normal Mean Measurements (cm)

Age	*AP diameter*	*Transverse*	*Craniocaudal*
0-10 yr	2.52 ± 0.82	3.13 ± 0.85	3.53 ± 0.99
10-20 yr	2.56 ± 0.88	3.05 ± 1.17	4.99 ± 1.25
20-30 yr	2.38 ± 0.72	2.87 ± 0.86	5.38 ± 1.80

Choanal Air Space

Normal Value (mm)

Age	Size (mm)
Newborn	6.7 ± 1.70
0-2 yr	7.0 ± 1.65
8-10 yr	9.1 ± 1.70
14-16 yr	10.7 ± 1.70
18-20 yr	11.8 ± 1.65

CHOANAL ATRESIA

Findings on CT in < 2 yr old child -
   Posterior choanae narrowes to a width of <3.4 mm

Orbit Muscles Measurements

Normal values are-
- Superior oblique   2.4 ± 0.4 mm
- Lateral rectus   2.9 ± 0.6 mm
- Superior rectus   3.8 ± 0.7 mm
- Medial rectus   4.1 ± 0.5 mm
- Inferior rectus   4.9 ± 0.8 mm

Optic Nerve Sheath

- Waist   4.2 ± 0.6 mm
- Retrobulbar   5.5 ± 0.8 mm

Superior Ophthalmic Vein

- On coronal CT   2.7 ± 1.0 mm
- On axial CT   1.8 ± 0.5 mm

Globe Position

Normally eye ball is situated 9.9 ± 1.7 mm behind interzygomatic line.

Proptosis—When globe protrusion >21 mm anterior to interzygomatic line on axial scans at level of lens

Eyeball

Normal diameter in adult—around 2.5 cm

Macrophthalmia—(Diameter > 2.5 cm)

Common Causes

- Buphthalmos
- Axial myopia
- Melanoma/Retinoblastoma/Metastasis
- Connective tissue disorder—Ehlers-Danlos syndrome
- Marfan syndrome

Microphthalmia

Total Axial length of globe - < 10 mm (At Birth)
                          - < 12 mm (> 1 yr)

Common Causes

- Congenital rubella
- Persistent hyperplastic vitreous
- Phthisis bulbi
- Trauma/surgery/radiation therapy

Chapter 7

Hepatobiliary System

GALLBLADDER

Normal measurements
Pediatric gallbladder length -

< 1 yr	- 1.5-3 cm
>1 yr	- 3-7 cm

Adult gallbladder-

Length	- 7-10 cm
Width	- 2 - 3.5 cm

SMALL GALLBLADDER

Common Causes

- Postprandial
- Chronic cholecystitis
- Congenital hypoplasia
- Cystic fibrosis.

CHOLECYSTOMEGALY

Refers to Enlarged Gallbladder - When length > 10 cm, width > 3.5 cm

Common Causes

- Cholelithiasis
- Cystic duct obstruction
- Cholecystitis with cholelithiasis
- Pancreatitis
- Typhoid fever, ascariasis infection
- Alcoholism
- Diabetes mellitus
- Prolonged fasting/Dehydration/total parenteral nutrition

- Normal in few individuals
- Sepsis.

Gallbladder Stone (Fig. 7.1)

Stones > 5 mm — give shadow and are echogenic

Stones < 5 mm—usually does not shadow, but still appear echogenic

Diffuse Gallbladder Wall Thickening

Normal wall thickness—2-3 mm

Abnormal—when anterior wall of gallbladder measures >3 mm

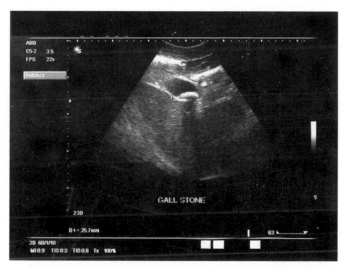

Fig. 7.1: Gallbladder stone with acoustic shadowing

Common causes are
- A/c/ch. cholecystitis
- Sepsis
- Gallbladder carcinoma
- Hepatitis, Cirrhosis
- Ascites
- Right heart failure
- Renal failure
- Contracted after eating

Polypoid Mass of Gallbladder

Malignant criteria
- Usually >10 mm in size
- Single in number
- Rapid change in size on follow-up sonography
- Age >60 yr

Benign criteria
- Usually <10 mm in size
- Multiple
- No change in size on follow up sonography.

Pancreas

Normal AP diameter
- Head = < 3 cm
- Body = < 2 cm
- Tail = < 2.5 cm

Note - Size decreases with age

Main Pancreatic Duct of Wirsung
- Measures 1-2 mm in diameter, smoothly outlined

- Receives 20-35 tributaries/side branches that enter at right angles
- In normal pancreatic duct—walls are smooth, lumen is clear and walls maintain their parallel course
- When duct is dilated—walls become irregular.

UNILOCULAR PANCREATIC CYST

When cyst measures <3 cm in diameter, it is almost always benign and should be followed at 6-month intervals for 3 years. For example,
- Pseudocyst
- Lymphoepithelial cyst
- Unilocular serous cystadenoma

Microcystic Lesion of Pancreas

It refers to pancreatic lesion with >6 cysts and each cyst measures <2 cm in size, e.g. serous cystadenoma

Macrocystic Lesion of Pancreas

It refers to multilocular cyst, and each compartment measures >2 cm in size.

For example, mucinous cystic neoplasm.

Indication for Pancreatic Pseudocyst Drainage

Persistence of pseudocyst >5 cm
- Persistence > 6 weeks
- Increasing size of cyst on follow-up
- Pain and suspected infection
- Biliary/gastrointestinal obstruction

Pancreatic Necrosis

It refers to focal/diffuse area of non viable pancreatic parenchyma

Radiological Measurement Findings on Contrast CT

Focal/diffuse well-marginated zone of unenhanced pancreatic parenchyma involving >30% or > 3 cm of the pancreatic gland.

SPLEEN (FIG. 7.2)

Normal Length
- 0-3 months of age—< 6.0 cm
- Children—5.7 + 0.31 × age (in yrs)

Length in Pediatric Age Group (cm)

Normal range	Male	Female
0-4 yrs -	5.9 ± 1.18	5.77 ± 1.21
5-9 yrs -	7.8 ± 1.28	7.48 ± 1.21
10-14 yrs -	9.10 ± 1.41	8.76 ± 1.10

Adults - 11 cm length
- 7 cm anteroposterior diameter
- 4 cm thickness

Splenomegaly

Criteria

- When size is more than normal range,
- Also look for any rotundness—i.e. The original crescentric configuration with its pointed poles gets lost and the poles become rounded or blunted

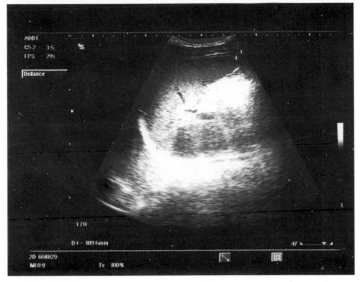

Fig. 7.2: Normal spleen

- Most commonly used method is—*eyeball technique*, i.e. if it looks big, it is big.

Common causes are
- Portal hypertension
- Cirrhosis
- Heart failure
- Lymphoma, leukemia, metastases
- Mucopolysaccharidoses
- Typhoid fever, TB, syphilis, viral hepatitis, malaria, kala azar
- Hereditary spherocytosis

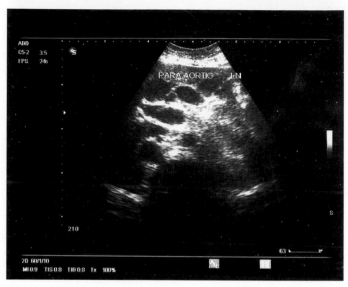

Fig. 7.3: Pre-and para-aortic lymphadenopathy

Lymph Nodes (Fig. 7.3)

Normal abdomen lymph node meas—7–10 mm in length.

Benign Lymph Node

Common features
- Shape— ovoid
- L/T ratio—> 2, where L- longitudinal diameter, T- transverse diameter (width)
- *Hilar sign*—hyperechoic hilar structure in the centre of the enlarged lymph node surrounded by a hypoechoic periphery.

Common causes are-
- – Viral hepatitis
- – Pancreatitis
- – Cholangitis
- – Cholecystitis
- Vascularity—centred in the hilus

Malignant Lymph Node

Common features are-
- Shape   spherical
- L/T ratio   1
- Hilar sign   absent
- Vascularity   branching/diffuse pattern

Liver Normal Size (Fig. 7.4)

In Adult

- *Along midclavicular line* (vertical/craniocaudad axis)-
  Normal < 13 cm
  Indeterminate 13- 15.5 cm
  Hepatomegaly > 15.5
- *Along prerenal line* <14 cm
- *Along preaortic line* <10 cm
- *Inferior marginal angle* of right hepatic lobe— < 45%
  In Hepatomegaly > 45 %
- *Lateral marginal angle* of left lobe should be— < 30 %
  In Hepatomegaly— > 30%
- *Caudate lobe*   < 5 cm craniocaudally
                   < 2.5 cm anteroposteriorly

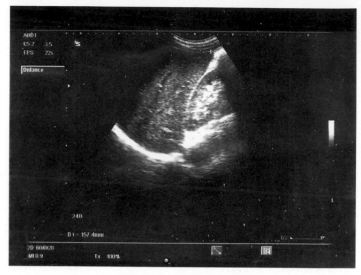

Fig. 7.4: Hepatomegaly

In Children

Right hepatic lobe should not extend below right costal margin.

In Young Infant

Right hepatic lobe should not extend >1 cm below right costal margin.

POLYCYSTIC LIVER DISEASE

Radiological measurement findings—enlarged diffusely cystic liver (cysts of 1 mm to12 cm in diameter)
• ± diffuse dilatation of intra- and extrahepatic bile ducts
• calcifications of cyst walls.

Commonly associated with—Polycystic kidney disease

Clinically present as—Upper abdominal pain and distension.

CIRRHOSIS

Types

- *Micronodular cirrhosis* (size of nodule <3 mm)—common causes are biliary obstruction, alcoholism and hemochromatosis.
- *Macronodular cirrhosis (size of nodule 3-15 mm or up to several cm)* common causes are Wilson's disease, chronic viral hepatitis, alpha-1 antitrypsin deficiency.

Radiological Measurement Findings

It can present as enlarged (in early stage)/normal/shrunken liver

- Shrinkage of left lobe segments 4a, 4b and right lobe segments 5-8
- Concomitant hypertrophy of caudate lobe (segment 1), left lobe segments 2 and 3
- Ratio of width of caudate to right lobe > 0.65 on transverse images
- Widened porta hepatis and interlobar fissure
- Diameter of quadrate lobe (segment 4) <30 mm
- Signs of portal hypertension.

Hydatid Disease—(Echinococcus Granulosous)

Normal length	- 3-6 mm
Definitive host	- Dog
Intermediate host	- Humans, sheep, cattle

Features

Living embryos form slow growing cyst.

Cyst wall has three layers
- *Ectocyst*—usually 1 mm thick, may get calcify
- *Pericyst*—dense connective tissue capsule around the cyst formed by host
- *Endocyst*—inner layer.

Cavernous Hemangioma of Liver

- Most common benign liver tumor, usually < 4 cm
- Giant cavernous hemangioma—when size is > 4 cm.

Commonly associated with:
Focal nodular hyperplasia/Hemangiomas in other organs

Criteria for Liver Transplant in Early HCC Cases

- No leison should be > 5 cm in diameter or
- No more than 3 leisons of > 3 cm diameter.

Maximum Normal Cross-sectional Diameter of Portal Vein (Fig. 7.5)

- Adult - 13.0 mm
- 10-20 yr - 10.0 mm
- <10 yr - 8.5 mm

Portal Hypertension

Radiological measurement findings are
- Portal vein ≥ 15 mm
- Increased echogenicity and thickening of portal vein walls
- Superior mesentric vein and splenic vein >10 mm;
- Coronary vein > 4 mm;

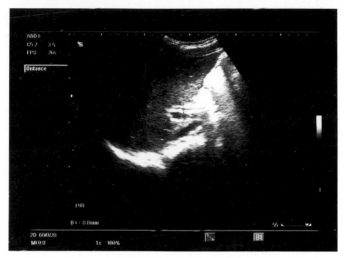

Fig. 7.5: Normal portal vein

- Recanalized umbilical vein >3 mm
- Loss of respiratory increase of splanchnic vein diameters of <20%
- Ascites, splenomegaly
- Siderotic Gamma-Gandy nodules refers to small foci of perifollicular and trabecular 3-8-mm size hemorrhage.

Common causes are
- Cirrhosis /Hepatitis
- Portal vein thrombosis/portal vein compression by tumor, trauma
- Budd-Chiari syndrome
- Wilson's disease
- Alpha-1 antitrypsin deficiency
- Sickle cell disease.

BILE DUCTS

Cystic Duct

Normal Measurements
Length - 1-2 cm
Diameter - 1.8 mm

Normal Size of CBD
Neonates - <1 mm
Up to 1 yr - <2 mm
older children - <4 mm

Adolescents and adults
- ≤ 5 mm - normal
- 6-7 mm - equivocal
- ≥ 8 mm - dilated

Note - In patient >70 years of age add 1 mm/decade
- In postcholecystectomy patients up to 8 mm is normal

- *CHD at porta hepatis and CBD in head of pancreas—5 mm*
- *Right intrahepatic bile duct just proximal to CHD—2-3 mm* or <40% of diameter of accompanying portal vein.

Hepatic Veins

- Normal diameter at periphery— < 6 mm
- Right heart decompensation— >6 mm.

Chapter 8

Obstetrics

FETAL PARAMETERS

Gestational SAC (GS)

It refers to the average of 3 diameters (length, AP, width) of anechoic space within sac walls.

- On transabdominal scan—identified as early as 5 weeks MA.
- Used for dating between 6 and 12 weeks MA
- EGA [in wks] = (GS [mm] + 25.43) ÷ 7.02

Gestational Sac and Corresponding Menstrual Age

- 10 mm   - 5 wk   ± 1 wk
- 13 mm   - 5 wk 5 days   ± 1 wk
- 17 mm   - 6 wk   ± 1 wk
- 20 mm   - 6 wk 5 days   ± 1 wk
- 60 mm   - 12 wk   ± 1 wk

Embryo

Earliest visualization on TVS - 5.4 weeks MA at CRL of 1.2 mm

Visualization of Embryo Versus Gestational SAC

- *On transvaginal scan*   - 100% visualization of embryo if gestational sac measures ≥ 12 mm
- *On transabdominal scan*   - 100% visualization of embryo if gestational sac measures ≥ 27 mm

Failed pregnancy—Non-visualization of embryo when mean gestational sac size measures ≥ 18 mm.

Yolk Sac

- It is the site of earliest blood cell formation
- Time of formation—at around 28 days—menstrual age
- First visible structure within gestational sac
- Definite visualization on TVS—at 5.5 weeks of MA
- Definite visualization on transabdominal scan- at 7 weeks of MA.

Mean Size

1.0 mm - 4.7 weeks MA
2.0 mm - 5.6 weeks MA
3.0 mm - 7.1 weeks MA
4.0 mm - 10 weeks MA
Finally disappears - around 12 weeks MA

Significance

At 10 weeks of gestation—if yolk sac diameter is < 3 mm or > 7 mm, it implies an increased risk for developmental anomalies.

Umbilical Cord (Fig. 8.1)

- Umbilical cord grows until end of 2nd trimester:
- Normal length–50-60 cm, and diameter—1-2 cm
- Contents—two umbilical arteries, 1 umbilical vein (Mickey-Mouse Sign)

Cardiac Activity of Embryo

Embryo heart begins to contract at a CRL of 1.5-3 mm (22 days GA)

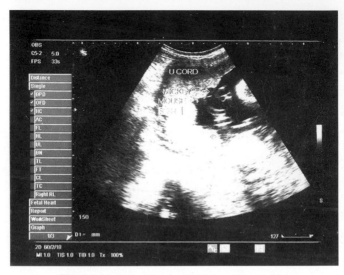

Fig. 8.1: Umbilical Cord with Mickey-Mouse Sign

- *Definite visualization on transabdominal scan*—when mean sac diameter measures 25 mm or at 55 days of gestational age
- *Definite visualization of cardiac activity on TVS*—when mean sac diameter measures 16 mm or at 46 days of Gestational age.

Normal Heart Rate in Early Pregnancy

Heart Rate (Bpm)—2.6 x MSD (mm) + 82

Normal Range
6 weeks — 90- 131 (bpm)
7 weeks — 123-185 (bpm)
8 weeks — 139-181 (bpm)

FETAL AGE ESTIMATION

It involves the measurement of following parameters:

Femur Measurement

- Measurement are made from one end to the other end
- Femur is easiest bone to recognize and measure
- A femur is short if it is more than 2 SD below the mean range
- If femur length is even smaller or 5 mm smaller than 2 SD, skeletal dysplasia is likely to be present.

Biparietal Diameter (BPD)

Best method of estimating GA when menstrual age is between 12-26 weeks.

Measurement plane—taken at the level when shape of skull is ovoid, thalami and cavum septi pellucidi seen interrupting the midline echo from falx cerebri measured from leading edge to leading edge of calvarial table at widest transaxial plane of skull, i.e. from outer table of proximal skull to inner table of distal skull.

Head Circumference (HC)

$HC = (BPD + FOD) \times 1.57$
FOD—fronto-occipito diameter
BPD—biparietal diameter

Significance

- *HC too small*—Commonly seen in synostosis, anencephaly, cerebral infarction

- *HC too large*—Commonly seen in hydrocephalus, intracranial hemorrhage, tumor

Fetal Cerebellum

Normal values

Transcerebellar diameter (mm)	Gestational age (week)
14	15.3
15	16.0
16	16.8
17	17.6
18	18.3
19	19.1
20	19.9
21	20.7
22	21.5
23	22.2
24	23.0

Abdominal Circumference (AC)

Measurement plane—AC is taken at level of umbilical part of left portal vein (hockey stick appearance);
- It is measured from outer edge to outer edge of soft tissues.
- It allows evaluation of head-to-body disproportion, i.e. detects IUGR.
- It is a good predictor of fetal weight.

Significance

- *AC too small* (less than 5th percentile)—Commonly seen in diaphragmatic hernia, gastroschisis, renal agenesis, omphalocele

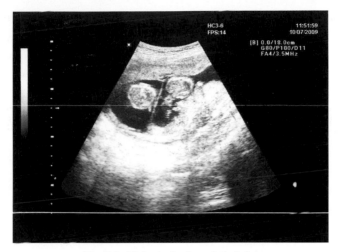

Fig. 8.2: Dichorionic diamniotic twins

- *AC too large* (more than 95th percentile)—Commonly seen in hepatosplenomegaly, abdominal tumor, GIT obstructions, obstructive uropathy, ascites.

Dichorionic Diamniotic Twins (Fig. 8.2)

Common Measurement Findings

Membrane thickness measures >2 mm, due to 2 separate chorionic sacs and 2 separate amniotic sacs, separate fused/ unfused placentas.

Monochorionic Twins

Common featu res are:
- Monochorionic membrane (two layers of amnion <1 mm).
- Absence of membrane suggests a monoamniotic monochorionic twin pregnancy.

Inevitable Abortion (Abortion in Progress)

In this condition, gestational sac with embryo have become detached from implantation site which leads to spontaneous abortion within next few hours.

Common **USG** findings are—cervix is dilated and measures >3 cm gestational sac is located low within uterus with progressive migration of sac toward/into cervical canal.

Clinical Triad
- Persistent painful uterine contractions
- Bleeding >7 days
- Rupture of membranes.

Nonviability of Fetus, Criteria on Transvaginal Scan

- No yolk sac with GS measurement of 6-9 mm
- No cardiac activity with GS of ≥ 9 mm
- Thinning of choriodecidual reaction with hypoechoic clefts, distorted sac configuration
- *Normal USG Milestones Not Met as Expected*
- Gestational sac first identifiable ≥ 5.0 week
- Yolk sac first identifiable ≥ 5.5 week
- Embryo and FHM first identifiable ≥ 6.0 week

Blighted Ovum (An Embryonic Pregnancy)

It refers to abnormal intrauterine pregnancy with developmental arrest prior to formation of embryo.

*Common **USG** findings are*
- Gestational sac is empty (>6.5 weeks MA), shape is distorted and size is small
- Decidual reaction is irregular, weakly echogenic, measures < 2 mm

- Yolk sac identified without embryo
- On serial scans—Gestational sac fails to grow by >0.6 mm/day and vanishing yolk sac.

On Transabdominal USG

- Gestational sac size ≥ 20 mm of mean diameter without yolk sac
- Gestational sac size ≥ 25 mm of mean diameter without embryo.

Incomplete Abortion (Retained Products of Conception)

In this condition, portion of placental or fetal tissue remains within uterus.

*Common **USG** findings are:*
- Endometrium thickness is >5 mm
- Gestational sac shows dead fetus/collection
- Gestational sac is irregular/angulated, small in size, contains amorphous echogenic material
- Choriodecidual reaction is ragged disrupted
- Subchorionic fluid ± hemorrhage
  Clinically present as—continued genital bleeding, patulous cervix.

Missed Abortion

Refers to dead conceptus within uterine cavity of gestational age ≥ 8 weeks, occurring prior to 28 weeks MA.

Common USG findings are:
- Cardiac activity is absent in embryo with CRL >5 mm (on TVS)/CRL >9 mm (on transabdominal scan)
- *Gestation age not corresponding to menstrual age*

- Gestational sac >20 mm in diameter without yolk sac
- Gestational sac >25 mm in diameter without an embryo
- Irregular/discontinuous/thin (2 mm) choriodecidual reaction
- Subchorionic collection
- Sac appears—crenated irregular with debris within gestational sac.

Normal Cervical Length in Gravid Uterus

On Transabdominal Scan

1st trimester	53 ± 17 mm
2nd trimester	44 ± 14 mm
3rd trimester	40 ± 10 mm

Incompetent Cervix

It refers to gaping of cervix usually developing during 2nd trimester/early 3rd trimester.
Risk factors—cervical trauma (cauterization, D and C)

USG findings are:
- Cervix is shortened to <25 mm
- Cervical canal begins dilating at internal os and extends toward external os., with visualization of fetal parts within dilated endocervical canal
- Beaking/funneling of cervical canal, with bulging of membranes through external os.

Dilated Cervix

Commonly seen in:
- Incompetent cervix
- Premature labor
- Inevitable abortion

Intrauterine Growth Retardation

Types—symmetric/asymmetric/mixed

Symmetric IUGR

Following are the features—early-insult IUGR (decreased cell-number IUGR), occurs before 26 wks GA, there is *proportionate* decrease in HC and AC, maintaining normal HC ÷ AC ratios, fetal weight measures <10th percentile for age.

Asymmetric IUGR

Following are the features—late-onset IUGR (decreased cell-size IUGR) occurs after 26 weeks GA, there is *disproportionate* decrease in fetal measurements due to uteroplacental insufficiency with preferential shunting of blood to fetal brain occurring.
• HC ÷AC and FL ÷ AC ratios are high
• AC >2 SD below the mean for age – highly suspicious for IUGR
• AC >3 SD below mean for age diagnostic for IUGR
• Umbilical artery S/D ratio is increased
• Amniotic fluid volume is decreased.

Macrosomia

When fetus is large for gestational age with EFW >4,000 g at term / >90th percentile for age
• AC >3 SD above the mean for age
• HC ÷ AC ratio and FL ÷ AC ratio is low
• Greater than expected interval growth
• Thigh circumference is increased
• FL ÷ thigh circumference ratio is low
• Polyhydramnios

Uterus Large-for-Dates

Commonly seen in:
- Hydatidiform mole
- Polyhydramnios
- Fetal macrosomia
- Multiple gestation pregnancy
- Inaccurate menstrual history

Amniotic Fluid Index (AFI)

Used to assess amniotic fluid volume.

It refers to the sum of vertical depths of largest clear amniotic fluid pockets (free of umbilical cord and fetal parts) in the 4 uterine quadrants.

Commonly measured in cm.

Method—Patient lies supine, uterus viewed as 4 equal quadrants, transducer should be perpendicular to plane of floor and aligned longitudinally with patient's spine.

Twin AFI—calculated by same procedure as in single pregnancy.

Amniotic Fluid Volume in First Trimester

Formula- $4/3\Omega \times$ (AP diameter$/2 \times$ transverse diam$/2 \times$ longitudinal diam$/2$)

Where AP, transverse and longitudinal are the gestational sac diameter

Normal Range

Gestational age	*Amniotic fluid volume (ml)*
8 weeks	0.9- 11.2

9 weeks	5.2- 28.6
10 weeks	9.3- 37.8
11 weeks	23.8- 86
12 weeks	27.4- 90

Variations in AFI

Oligohydramnios

Criteria—When amniotic fluid volume measures <500 ml at term
- AFI is ≤ 7 cm
- Single largest pocket ≤ 2 cm in vertical direction.

Common causes are:
Premature rupture of membranes (most common)/, Postmaturity renal agenesis/dysgenesis, prune belly syndrome, infantile polycystic kidney disease, urethral atresia, posterior urethral valves, cloacal anomalies, IUGR/ fetus demise.

Polyhydramnios

Criteria—When amniotic fluid volume measures > 1500- 2000 ml at term
- AFI is ≥ 20- 24 cm
- Single largest pocket measures >8 cm
Common causes are:
- Fetal—High intestinal/esophageal/tracheal atresias obstruction of bowel hydranencephaly, anencephaly, holoprosencephaly, ventriculomegaly, encephalocele, agenesis of corpus callosum, microcephaly
  - Trisomy 13, 18, 21
  - Ventricular septal defect

- – Unilateral uretropelvic junction obstruction, unilateral multicystic dysplastic kidney.
- *Maternal*—Rh-incompatibility, diabetes
- *Idiopathic*

BPP SCORE—BIOPHYSICAL PROFILE SCORE

Purpose—for assessment of fetal well-being.

It includes the following parameters—

- *Quantitative amniotic fluid volume*—1 pocket of fluid measuring 2 cm in vertical axis.
- *Fetal posture and fetal tone*—One episode of active extension with return to flexion of fetal limbs or trunk, opening and closing of hand also considered normal tone.
- *Fetal breathing movement*—One episode of > 30 of fetal breathing movement in 30 min or less
- *Fetal movement*—3 discrete body/limb movements in 30 min or less
- *Reactive fetal heart (NST)*—Two episodes of acceleration of > 15 bpm and > 15 associated with fetal movement in 20 min

If above findings are present then score of 2/2 for each variable, and if abnormal findings then score of 0/2 for each variable.

Placentomegaly

It refers to increase in placenta thickness measuring >5 cm, in sections obtained at right angles to long axis of placenta.

Common causes are:

- *Fetal*—Fetal hydrops, hemolytic disease of the newborn, chromosomal abnormality, umbilical vein obstruction, fetomaternal hemorrhage.

- *Maternal*—Anemia, diabetes, syphilis.
- *Placenta*—Molar pregnancy, Chorioangioma, Intra-placental hemorrhage.

Decrease in Placental Size

Common causes are:
- IUGR
- Preeclampsia
- Chromosomal abnormality

Ventricles

- Normal width of 3rd ventricle: <3.5 mm (any gestational age).
- Normal width of ventricular atrium <10 mm.

Fetal Ventriculomegaly

Width of ventricular atrium >10 mm, dangling choroid plexus.

Common causes are:
- Encephalocele
- Spina bifida
- Holoprosencephaly
- Dandy-Walker malformation
- Agenesis of corpus callosum.

Fetal Hydrocepalus

Ventricle hemisphere ratio—It refers to the ratio of frontal/occipital horn diameter to the hemispheric diameter.

Normal ratio   < 0.5
In hydrocephalus   > 0.5

Cisterna Magna

Diameter of Cisterna Magna

- Measured from inner margin of occiput to vermis cerebelli:
- Normal size between 15-25 weeks MA is 2-10 mm.

Large Cisterna Magna

Commonly seen in:
- *Megacisterna magna*—cerebellum and vermis remain intact
- Dandy-Walker syndrome (with vermian agenesis) arachnoid cyst
- Cerebellar hypoplasia

Small Cisterna Magna

Commonly seen in-
- Occipital cephalocele
- Chiari II malformation
- Severe hydrocephalus

Nuchal Skin Thickening

Synonyms—Nuchal Fullness/Edema/Sonolucency

It refers to skin thickening of posterior neck measured between calvarium and dorsal skin margin.

Plane—Image taken in transcerebellar diameter view, i.e. at axial plane that includes cavum septi pellucidi, cisterna magna and cerebellar hemisphere.

Significance—Septations within nuchal translucency carries a 20 to 200-fold risk for chromosomal anomalies compared with normal.

- Nuchal skin thickening is 99% specific for detection of Down's syndrome.
- *Abnormal values are:*
    ≥ 3 mm during 9-13 weeks MA
    ≥ 5 mm during 14- 21 weeks MA
    ≥ 6 mm during 19- 24 weeks MA.

Common causes are:
- Down's syndrome
- Turner syndrome
- XYY/XXX syndrome
- Klippel-Feil syndrome
- Trisomy 18.

NUCHAL TRANSLUCENCY

It refers to measurement of space between spine and overlying skin on midsagittal view ideal time to look for nuchal translucency: 10w3d to 13w6d of EGA.

Abnormal if values are:
≥ 5 mm during 14-18 weeks
≥ 6 mm during 19-24 weeks
Marker for—Down syndrome

BOWEL OBSTRUCTION IN FETUS

OB-USG *measurement findings:*
Multiple distended bowel loops >7 mm in diameter, increased peristalsis

Common causes are:
- Meconium ileus
- Intussusception

- Intestinal atresia/stenosis
- Volvulus.

Fetal Hydronephrosis

OB USG measurement findings:
When AP diameter of renal pelvis is:
- at 15-20 weeks   > 5 mm
- at 20-30 weeks   ≥ 8 mm
- at >30 weeks   ≥ 10 mm

Common causes are:

- Ectopic ureterocele
- Ureteropelvic junction obstruction
- Posterior/anterior urethral valves
- Prune belly syndrome
- Ureteral and vesicoureteric junction obstruction
- Congenital urethral strictures
- Severe vesicoureteral reflux.

Chapter 9

Gynecology

NORMAL UTERINE SIZE

Neonate Uterus

- Fundal width   - 0.8 -2 .1 cm
- Cervical width   - 0.8- 2.2 cm
- Length   - 2.3- 4.6 cm

Infantile Uterus—infancy till 7 years age

- Fundal width   - 0.4-1.0 cm
- Cervical width   - 0.6-1.0 cm
- Length   - 2.5-3.3 cm

Presuberty Uterus

- Mean length of 4.3 cm
- Fundocervical ratio of 1:1

Postpuberty Uterus

Fundocervical ratio of 2:1 to 3 :1

In multiparous

AP	- 3-4 cm
Trans	- 3-5 cm
Length	- 6-11 cm

In nulliparous

AP	- 3 cm
Trans	- 4.5-5.5
Length	- 5-8 cm

Note

Primi paras increases the normal size by   - 1 cm
Multi paras increases the normal size by   - 2 cm

Postmenopausal Uterus

- Cervix occupies 1/3 of uterine length
- AP   - 2 cm
- Length - 3.5- 6.5 cm
- Trans   - 1.2-1.8 cm.

Diffuse Uterine Enlargement

Common causes are:
- Diffuse fibroid
- Adenomyosis
- Endometrial carcinoma

UTERUS DEVELOPMENTAL ANOMALIES

Uterus Bicornis/Bicornuate Uterus (Fig. 9.1)

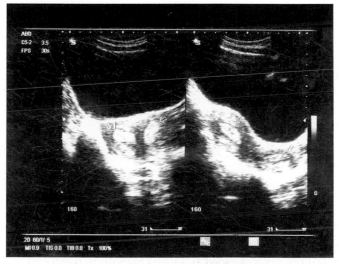

Fig. 9.1: Bicornuate Uterus

Types

a. Bicornis bicollis—complete separation of uterine horns with division down to internal os

b. Bicornis unicollis— partial separation of uterine horns common **MRI** findings are:
  - intercornual distance >4 cm
  - intercornual angle of >75-105°
  - external uterine fundal contour shows concave surface depression >2 cm, deep large fundal cleft, fusiform shape of each uterine horn with lateral convex margins elongation and widening of cervical canal and isthmus.

Clinically present as:
- Repeated spontaneous abortions
- Premature rupture of membranes/premature labor.

Septate Uterus

*Common **MRI** findings are:*
- Intercornual angle of ≤ 75°
- External fundal contour ≤ 1 cm, flat/minimally indented
- Endometrial canals completely separated by tissue isoechoic to myometrium extending into endocervical canal.

Types

- *Uterus subseptus*—partial septum involving endometrial canal
- *Uterus septus*—complete septum which extends till internal os

Displaced Intrauterine Device

- If IUD and fundus distance is > 2 cm,
- It suggests displaced IUD and is close to the cervix, this leads to less reliable contraceptive effect.

VAGINA

In posthysterectomy patients ,
- Normal AP diameter of vaginal cuff — < 2.1 cm
- Suspect malignancy when cuff size — > 2.1 cm.

Endometrium

Endometrium thickness—Refers to AP diameter of both apposed endometrial layers, excluding intrauterine fluid

Plane of measurement—Taken at the level of the uterine fundus, midline long-axis image of uterus
Note: In large body habitus females measurements increase by 1-2 mm:

Endometrium in different phases—

Menstrual Phase (Days 1-5)

Features	-	Interrupted thin echogenic line of central interface
Thickness	-	1-4 mm

Proliferative Phase (Days 6-14)

Features	- thickened hypochoic endometrium
Thickness	- 5-7 mm

Periovulatory Phase (Day 14)

Features	- triple ring sign (multilayered endometrium)
Thickness	- up to 11 mm

Secretory Phase (Days 15-28)

Features	- markedly echogenic thick endometrium
Thickness	- up to 14 mm

Normal Postpartum Endometrium

Features—small echogenic foci of clot/retained membranes/debris endometrial cavity measures<20 mm in diameter.

Postmenopausal Endometrium

- *No hormonal replacement therapy*—bilayer thickness of <5 mm with a homogeneous echogenic endometrium
- *With hormonal replacement therapy*—endometrial thickness may increase to 15 mm.

Endometrial Hyperplasia

Commonly seen in:
- Peripostmenopausal women
- Focal/diffuse endometrial thickening >5-6 mm
- Formation of polyps of up to 5 cm.

Focally Thickened Endometrium

Commonly seen in
- Primary carcinoma of the endometrium
  Risk factors-obesity, diabetes, nulliparity, exposure to unopposed estrogen, hypertension,
  10% cancer rate with endometrial thickness of 6-15 mm
  50% cancer rate with endometrial thickness of >15 mm
- Endometrial polyp
- Metastatic carcinoma
- Focal adenomyoma

Fallopian Tube

Location - Superior aspect of broad ligament
Normal Length - 7-12 cm

Parts

- *Ampullary portion*—refers to widened region near ovary
- *Isthmic portion*—long narrow part between interstitial and ampullary end
- Interstitial/cornual portion—short segment that traverses muscular wall of the uterus.

Ovarian Size

Ovarian volume = Length × Width × Height × 0.523

<3 months	:	1.06-3.56 cc
4-12 months	:	up to 2.7 cc
1 year	:	1.05 ± 0.7 cc
2-6 years	:	≤ 1.0 ± 0.4 cc
6-10 years	:	2-2.3 cc
11-12 years	:	2-4 cc
After puberty	:	2.5-20cc

Postmenopausal Ovary

Normal range- 1.2 – 5.8 cc
Abnormal:
- If ≥ 8 cc
- If one side volume is twice that of opposite side

Postmenopausal Cysts

Common features are:
- Small anechoic, well defined, round, cyst
- *Size*—usually < 3 cm diam
- *Common in* —post hysterectomy women
- Suggested follow up, usually resolves with time.

Surgery recommended
- If > 5 cm in size
- Contains nodules/septations.

Follicular Cyst

Common features are–
- When mature follicle fails to ovulate/involute
- *Size* 1-20 cm
- *Clinically*—asymptomatic, usually unilateral and regress spontaneously.

Ovarian Hyperstimulation Syndrome

Refers to complication of ovulation induction characterized by three forms—mild/moderate/severe
Mild form—ovaries enlarged and measures < 5 cm in diameter, lower abdomen pain.

Severe form—Common Features

- Associated with weight gain, distention and severe abdomen pain
- Ovarian diameter measures > 10 cm
- Contains multiple, large, thin walled cysts
- Associated with-ascites and pleural effusions.

Ovarian Cycle

Follicular Phase–days 1-14
- Unstimulated follicles measure <2 mm in size
- Stimulated follicles grow >2 mm in size, 2-3 follicles in each ovary of day 4 enlarge subsequently to approxi–mately 10 mm

- Day 10-single dominant follicle of 8-12 mm (graafian follicle), it grows by 2 mm/day and finally by day 14, enlarges to 17-24 mm.

Ovulatory Phase— day 14

- Ie rupture of mature graafian follicle with extrusion of ovum
- Free fluid appears in pouch of Douglas

Luteal Phase— days 15-28

- Corpus luteum of menstruation –refers to round/ovoid bulging protrusion on one side of ovary, it has mean diameter of 10-25 mm, and hyperechoic 1-4-mm thick wall
- Corpus luteum atreticum–refers to involution and atrophy of corpus luteum on about 24th day of cycle.

Signs of Ovulatory Failure

- Continuous cystic enlargement up to 30-40 mm
- Development of internal echoes before 18 mm size.

Polycystic Ovarian Disease (PCOD)

Common **USG** *features are*—bilaterally enlarged ovaries >15 cc, hypo/iso echoic multiple (> 5) small cysts of 5-8 mm, usually located peripherally can also occur randomly through out ovary.

Note—In few % of cases, PCOD may be unilateral.

Clinically oligo/amenorrrhoea
      obesity
      hirsutism

Nabothian Cyst

USG findings are:
- Single or multiple cyst in cervix detected incidentally
- *Size*—varies from few mm to 4 cm
- *Association*—with healing chronic cervicitis.

Chapter 10

Musculoskeletal System

CONGENITAL DYSPLASIA OF HIP/DEVELOPMENTAL DYSPLASIA OF HIP (DDH) (Fig. 10.1)

It refers to deformity of acetabulum due to disrupted relationship between femoral head and acetabulum.

Important Radiologic lines on plain pelvis radiograph are:

- *Line of Hilgenreiner*—it is the line connecting superolateral margins of triradiate cartilage.

  Significance—in DDH unilateral shortening of vertical distance from femoral metaphysis to Hilgenreiner's line is seen.

- *Acetabular angle*—it refers to angle that lies between Hilgenreiner's line and a line drawn from most superolateral ossified edge of acetabulum.

  Significance—acetabular angle >30° strongly suggests dysplasia.

- *Perkin's line*—it refers to vertical line to Hilgenreiner's line through the lateral rim of acetabulum.

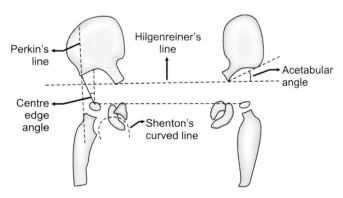

Fig. 10.1: AP pelvis radiograph

- *Shenton's curved line* — refers to arc formed by inferior surface of superior pubic ramus and medial surface of proximal femoral metaphysis to level of lesser trochanter. *Significance*—disruption of line seen DDH.
- *Center-edge angle*—refers to angle formed by line drawn from the acetabular edge to center of femoral head and second line perpendicular to line connecting centers of femoral heads.
  Significance— < 25° suggests femoral head instability.

ILIAC ANGLE AND INDEX (Fig. 10.2)

Radiograph—AP pelvis

Important Landmarks

Iliac Angle—line is drawn tangential to the most lateral margin of the iliac wing and iliac body, another line is drawn through the triradiate cartilage at the pelvic rim (y-y line), angle formed

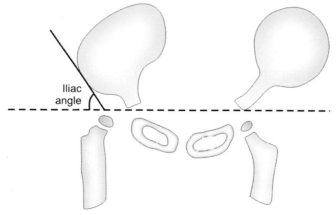

Fig. 10.2: AP pelvis radiograph

by intersecting of these lines is called iliac angle.

Normal Values

0-3 months	- 35°-58°
3-12 months	- 43°-67 °

Iliac index—This is the sum of both the iliac angles and the acetabular angles divided by 2.

Normal Values

0-3 months	- 48°-87 °
3-12 months	- 68°-97 °

Importance

Iliac index is most useful in the determination of Down's syndrome.

> *When value is:*
> < 60°   - Down's syndrome is probable
> 60-68°   - Syndrome is possible
> > 68°   - Syndrome is unlikely.

HIP JOINT SPACE WIDTH (Fig. 10.3)

Radiograph—AP hip

Important Landmarks

• *Axial joint space*—it is the space between the femoral head and acetabulum immediately lateral to the acetabular notch.

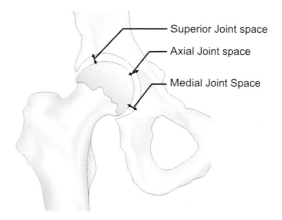

Fig. 10.3: Rt hip jt AP view

Significance—this space is decreased in degenerative arthritis, inflammatory arthritis.

• *Superior joint space*—it is the space between the superior most point on the convex articular surface of the femur and adjacent acetabular cortex.

Significance—this space is decreased in degenerative joint disease.

• *Medial joint space*—it is the space between the medial most surface of the femoral head and opposing acetabular surface.

Significance—this space is decreased in degenerative or inflammatory arthritis.

Widening of the hip joint spaces commonly seen in:

– Hip joint effusion
– Lateral shift of the femur.

Width Normal Values

Space	Width
Axial	3-7 mm
Superior	3-6 mm
Medial	4-13 mm

FEMORAL ANGLE (Femoral neck angle) (Fig. 10.4)

Radiograph—AP hip/pelvis.
Important landmarks—two lines are drawn through and parallel to the mid-axis of the femoral neck and femoral shaft. The angle obtained is then measured.

Normal Values for Femoral Angle

Minimum	- 120°
Maximum	- 130°

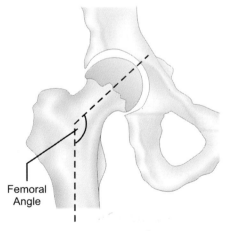

Fig. 10.4: Rt hip joint AP view

Significance

Coxa vara – when angle is < 120°
Coxa valga – when angle is > 130°

CARPAL ANGLE

It refers to the angle formed by intersection of tangents, to proximal row of carpal bones.
Normal value is — 130°

Increased Carpal Angle (When measures >139°)

Commonly seen in:
• Bone dysplasia with epiphyseal involvement
• Down's syndrome.

Decreased Carpal Angle (When measures <124°)

Commonly seen in:
• Hurler' syndrome
• Turner' syndrome
• Madelung deformity
• Morquio syndrome.

OSTEOPOROSIS

It refers to reduced bone mass of normal composition, secondary to osteoclastic and osteocytic resorption.

Dexa Score

Normal	>1
Osteopenia	≤ 1 and ≥ 2.5
Osteoporosis	≤ 2.5

Common causes are:
- Senile/postmenopausal/juvenile/adult osteoporosis
- Osteogenesis imperfecta
- Renal osteodystrophy
- Immobilization
- Radiation therapy.

Metacarpal Sign

It refers to relative shortening of 4th and 5th metacarpals

Important landmarks—when line drawn tangentially to distal end of the heads of 5th and 4th metacarpals, it Intersects head of 3rd metacarpal. Suggestive of positive metacarpal sign normally this line should pass distal to or just touch third metacarpal head.

Commonly seen in:
- Turner syndrome, Klinefelter syndrome
- Idiopathic
- Pseudohypoparathyroidism
- Sickle cell anemia
- Basal cell nevus syndrome
- Multiple epiphyseal dysplasia
- Melorheostosis
- Hereditary multiple exostoses.

Symphysis Pubis Width

Normal Values (mm)

Female   - 3.8- 6
Male   - 4.8-7.2

Widening of pubis symphysis seen in:
- Trauma
- Cleidocranial dysplasia
- Hyperparathyroidism
- Bladder exostrophy
- Inflammatory resorption (e.g. ankylosing spondylitis, gout).

Protrusio Acetabuli

It refers to bulging of acetabular floor into pelvis
Important landmarks—medial wall of acetabulum projects medially to ilioischial line by:
- > 6 mm (in females)
- > 3 mm (in males).

Common causes are:
- Paget disease
- Rheumatoid arthritis
- Osteomalacia
- Trauma
- Tuberculous arthritis.

Acetabular Depth (Fig. 10.5)

Radiograph—AP pelvis

Important landmarks—line is drawn from the superior margin of the pubic symphysis joint to the upper outer acetabular margin. The greatest distance from acetabular floor to this line is measured.

Normal Values for Acetabular Depth

Male   - 7-18 mm
Female   - 9-18 mm

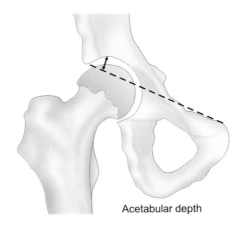

Acetabular depth

Fig. 10.5: Rt hip joint AP view

Decreased acetabular depth—Seen in degenerative joint disease of the hip.

Talo Calcaneal Angle

Refers to angle between talus and calcaneum, formed by lines drawn through mid transverse planes of calcaneum and talus.

Normal range
Infants and young children - 30-50°
In > 5 years   - 5-30°

Clubfoot/Talipes Equinovarus (Fig. 10.6)

It refers to severe congenital deformity characterized by:
- Heel varus (talocalcaneal angle of almost zero or even reversed on AP view with both bones parallel to each other).
- Mid talar and mid calcaneal line approach parallelism
- Both lines point lateral to normal position

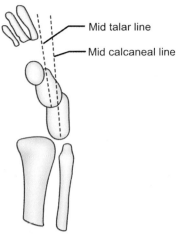

Fig. 10.6: Foot AP view

- Decreased calcaneal inclination angle/pitch (normally-20-30°)
- Metatarsus adductus (axis of 1st metatarsal deviated medially relative to axis of talus).

Common causes are:
- Spina bifida
- Neurofibromatosis
- Myelomeningocele.

Vertical Talus/Rocker-Bottom Foot

Radiological measurement findings:
- Heel equinus
- Vertically oriented talus with increased talocalcaneal angle on lateral view
- Dorsal navicular dislocation at talonavicular joint

Heelpad Thickening

It refers to increased heel pad thickening to >25 mm (normal value - < 21 mm)

Common causes are:
- Obesity
- Myxedema
- Peripheral edema
- Acromegaly.

ACHILLES TENDON

Origin—gastrocnemius and soleus muscle

Normal AP thickness   - 5-8 mm

In hypercholestremia patients   - 6-20 mm

Knee Joint Space Height

Normal range in adults (mm)

Lateral joint space - 6.30-7.58

Medial joint space - 5.58-7.15

Patellar Position

Radiograph—Lateral knee (semiflexed).

Important Landmarks

Patellar tendon length (PT)—it is the distance between the insertion points of the posterior tendon surface at the inferior patellar pole and the notch at the tibial tubercle.

Patellar length (PL)—refers to the greatest diagonal dimension between the superior and inferior poles.

Normal Measurements

PL and PT are usually equal to each other ± 20 %

Significance

Patella alta—When the patellar tendon length is >20 % greater than the patellar length.

Associated—with chondromalacia patellae.

Patella baja—(low riding patella) seen in—achondroplasia, polio, juvenile rheumatoid arthritis.

Calvarium Hemangiomas

Refers to round, osteolytic lesion with weblike/sunburst/spoke-wheel appearance of trabecular thickening:

Size—usually <4 cm

Common location—diploic space of frontal/parietal region

Benign Cortical Defect

Developmental intracortical bone defect

Site—metaphysis of long bone

Age—usually 1st-2nd decade

Size—usually <2 cm long

Appearance on radiograph—well-defined intracortical round/oval lucency with sclerotic margins.

Bone Island/Focal Sclerosis/Enostosis

Radiological Findings

Round or oval, solitary osteoblastic lesion with abrupt transition to surrounding normal trabecular bone.

Normal size—usually 2-10 mm in size;

Giant Bone Island—lesion >2 cm in longest axis

Rotary Subluxation of Scaphoid

It refers to tearing of interosseous ligaments of lunate, scaphoid and capitate

On PA view radiograph of hand
>4 mm gap is seen between scaphoid and lunate.

Flail Chest

It refers to fracture of >4 contiguous ribs

Cough Fracture

- Fractures commonly associated with excessive cough
- Common location–4-9th rib in anterior axillary line.

Jones Fracture

It refers to transverse fracture at base of 5th metatarsal bone at junction of metaphysis and diaphysis (>1.5 cm distal to proximal tip of metatarsal tuberosity).

Down' Syndrome—Trisomy 21st Chromosome

Radiological measurement findings in **OB USG**:

- Hypoplasia of middle phalanx of 5th digit resulting in clinodactyly
- Increased BPD/femur ratio
- Ratio of measured-to-expected humerus length ≤ 0.90
- Ratio of measured-to-expected femur length ≤ 0.91
- Mild fetal pyelectasis, polyhydramnios
- Frontal lobe shortening, small cerebellum, brachycephaly

- *Nuchal translucency*—refers to measurement of space between spine and overlying skin on midsagittal view ideal time to look for nuchal translucency:10w3d to 13w6d of EGA.

Values are:
- ≥ 5 mm during 14-18 weeks
- ≥ 6 mm during 19-24 weeks.

Marfan Synrome (Arachnodactyly)

Radiological measurement findings are:

Spine

- Expansion of sacral spinal canal
- Increased interpedicular distance
- Enlargement of sacral foramina
- Scoliosis/kyphoscoliosis
- Posterior scalloping.

Hand

- *Arachnodactyly*–refers to elongation of phalanges and metacarpals
- metacarpal index (averaging the 4 ratios of length of 2nd to 5th metacarpals divided by their respective middiaphyseal width)
- >9.4 in females and > 8.8 males.

Foot

- Disproportionate elongation of 1st digit of foot
- Pes planus, hallux valgus, clubfoot.

Turner Syndrome

Radiological measurement findings

Hand and Arm:

- Positive carpal sign of <117°
- *Positive metacarpal sign*—relative shortening of 3rd and 4th metacarpal
- *Drumstick distal phalanges*—slender shaft and large distal head
- *Phalangeal preponderance*—length of proximal and distal phalanx exceeds length of 4th metacarpal by >3 mm
- Shortening of 2nd and 5th middle phalanx
- *Madelung deformity*—shortening of ulna/absence of ulnar styloid process
  Skull—hypertelorism, basilar impression
  Foot—shortening of 1st, 4th, and 5th metatarsals
  Axial skeleton—hypoplasia of odontoid process and C1.

Glenohumeral Joint Space

Radiograph—AP shoulder with external rotation
Important landmarks—At the superior, middle and inferior aspects of the joint, measurements are made. There are combined and averaged.
Normal measurements—average joint space is 4-5 mm.

Decreased joint space commonly seen in:
- Degenerative arthritis
- Post-traumatic arthritis
- Calcium pyrophosphate dehydrate (CPPD) disease
- Widened joint space commonly seen in-
- Posterior humeral dislocation
- Acromegaly.

Acromiohumeral Joint Space

Radiograph—AP shoulder

Important landmarks—it refers to the distance between the inferior surface of the acromion and the articular cortex of the humeral head.

Normal range - 7 to 11 mm

Decreased joint space commonly seen in:
• Degenerative tendonitis
• Rotator cuff tear

Increased joint space commonly seen in:
• Trauma
• Joint effusion
• Dislocation
• Stroke
• Brachial plexus lesions (drooping shoulder).

Acromioclavicular Joint Space

Normal range:
Males   -   2.5 to 4.1 mm
Females   -   2.1 to 3.7 mm

• *Decreased joint space commonly seen in*—degenerative joint diseases.
• *Increased joint space commonly seen in* -
    – Trauma
    – Resorption 2° to osteolysis by hyperparathyroidism.

Chapter 11

Staging and Grading

STAGING OF CERVICAL CANCER

FIGO Stage	Description
0	Carcinoma *in situ* (before invasion)
I	Confined to cervix
IA	Preclinical invasive carcinoma
IA1	Microinvasion of stroma (<3 mm deep and <7 mm wide)
IA2	Tumor >3 mm but ≤ 7 mm horizontal spread
IB	Tumor larger than IA
IB1	≤ 4 cm
IB2	>4 cm
II	Extension beyond cervix but not to pelvic wall/lower one-third of vagina
IIA	Vaginal extension excluding lower 1/3
IIB	Parametrial invasion excepting pelvic sidewall
III	Extension to pelvic wall/lower third of vagina
IIIA	Invasion of lower 1/3 of vagina
IIIB	Pelvic side wall invasion and hydronephrosis
IV	Located outside true pelvis
IVA	Invasion of bladder/rectal mucosa
IVB	Spread to distant organs (para-aortic/inguinal nodes, intraperitoneal metastasis)

ENDOMETRIAL CANCER

FIGO stage	Description
0	*In situ*
Ia	Tumor limited to endometrium
Ib	Superficial invasion to <50% of myometrium
Ic	Deep invasion to more than half of myometrium
IIa	Endocervical glandular involvement only

IIb	Cervical stromal invasion
IIIa	Invasion of serosa/adnexa/peritoneal metastases
IIIb	Vaginal metastases
IIIc	Metastases to pelvic/para-aortic lymph nodes
IVa	Invasion of bladder/bowel mucosa
IVb	Distant metastases (lung, brain, bone) including intra-abdominal/inguinal lymph nodes

STAGING OF OVARIAN CANCER (FIGO SYSTEM) (FIG. 11.1)

Stage	*Description*
I	Limited to ovary
Ia	limited to one ovary
Ib	limited to both ovaries

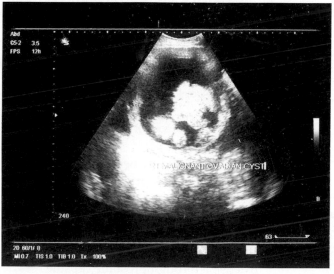

Fig. 11.1: Malignant ovarian cyst

Ic	Positive peritoneal lavage/ascites
II	Limited to pelvis
IIa	Involvement of uterus/fallopian tubes
IIb	Extension to other pelvic tissues
IIc	Positive peritoneal lavage/ascites
III	Limited to abdomen—intra-abdominal extension outside pelvis/retroperitoneal or inguinal nodes/extension to small bowel/ omentum
IIIa	Microscopic abdominal peritoneal seeding
IIIb	≤ 2 cm implants of abdominal peritoneum
IIIc	>2 cm implants of abdominal peritoneum
IV	Hematogenous disease (liver parenchyma)/ spread beyond abdomen

STAGING OF PROSTATE CANCER (AMERICAN JOINT COMMITTEE ON CANCER)

T0	No evidence of primary tumor
T1	Clinically inapparent nonpalpable nonvisible tumor
T1a	<3 microscopic foci of cancer/<5% of resected tissue
T1b	>3 microscopic foci of cancer/<5% of resected tissue
T1c	Tumor identified by needle biopsy
T2	Tumor clinically present and confined to prostate
T2a	Tumor 1.5 cm, normal tissue on 3 sides
T2b	Tumor <1.5 cm/in one lobe (unilateral)
T2c	Tumor involves both lobes (bilateral)
T3	Extension through prostatic capsule

T3a	Unilateral
T3b	Bilateral
T3c	Invasion of seminal vesicles
T4	Tumor fixed/invading adjacent structures other than seminal vesicles
T4a	Invasion of bladder neck, external sphincter, rectum
T4b	Invasion of levator anus muscle and/or fixed to pelvic wall
N	Involvement of regional lymph nodes
N1	Metastasis in a single node 2 cm
N2	Metastasis in a single node <2 and <5 cm/ multiple lymph nodes affected
N3	Metastasis in a lymph node 5 cm
M	Distant metastasis
M1a	Nonregional lymph nodes
M1b	Bone
M1c	Other site

STAGING OF WILMS' TUMOR

I	Tumor limited to kidney (renal capsule intact)
II	Local extension beyond renal capsule into perirenal tissue/renal vessels outside kidney/ lymph nodes
III	Not totally resectable (peritoneal implants, other than paraaortic nodes involved, invasion of vital structures)
IV	Hematogenous metastases/lymph node metastases outside abdomen or pelvis
V	Bilateral renal involvement at diagnosis

STAGING FOR RENAL CELL CARCINOMA

Robson Stage	TNM Class	Description
I		Tumor confined within renal capsule sharply defined convex interface with perirenal fat
	T1	Tumor <7 cm
	T2	Tumor 7 cm
II	T3	Extension into perinephric fat but confined to Gerota fascia irregular inter-face between tumor and fat
IIIA		Extension into renal vein or IVC
	T3b	Renal vein only
	T3c	Infradiaphragmatic IVC
	T4b	Supradiaphragmatic IVC
IIIB	N	Regional lymph nodes metastases
IIIC		Extension into renal vein and lymph nodes
IVA	T4a	Invasion of adjacent organs (other than ipsilateral adrenal)
IVB	M	Distant metastases

GRADING OF REFLUX IN CHILDREN

Grade I—reflux into distal ureter

Grade II—reflux into collecting system

Grade III—additional beginning uretral dilatation and caliceal clubbing

Grade IV—more pronounced uretral dilatation and caliceal clubbing

Grade V—marked caliceal clubbing and beginning parenchymal loss

GRADES OF VESICOURETERAL REFLUX (INTERNATIONAL REFLUX SYSTEM)

Grade I—reflux into ureter

Grade II—reflux into pelvicaliceal system (without caliceal dilatation/blunting)

Grade III—all of the above with mild dilatation of ureter and pelvicaliceal system distinct forniceal angles and papillary impressions

Grade IV—reflux into tortuous ureter and moderately dilated pelvicaliceal system, blunted forniceal angles and distinct papillary impressions

Grade V—reflux into markedly dilated and tortuous ureter with markedly dilated pelvicaliceal system obliteration of forniceal angles and papillary impressions.

CT/MRI FEATURES OF CYSTIC RENAL LESIONS BOSNIAK CLASSIFICATION

I   *Simple cyst:* Well-defined round mass of water attenuation hairline-thin imperceptible wall, no enhancement

II   *Minimally complicated cystic lesion:* Cluster of cysts/ septated cyst, minimal curvilinear calcification, minimally irregular wall high-density content

II^F *Follow-up lesion:* Hairline-thin septum/wall with perceived enhancement, intrarenal lesion >3 cm with high-density content

III *Complicated (surgical) lesion:* Hemorrhagic/infected cyst, MLCN, cystic neoplasm: Irregular thickened septa, measurable enhancement, coarse irregular calcification, irregular margin, multiloculated lesion, uniform wall thickening, nonenhancing nodular mass

IV   *Clearly malignant cystic lesion:* Large cystic/necrotic component, irregular wall thickening, solid enhancing elements.

STAGING OF TESTICULAR CANCER (AMERICAN JOINT COMMITTEE ON CANCER)

p^{TX} Primary tumor not available (no orchiectomy)

p^{T0} No primary tumor found

p^{Tis} Intratubular germ cell tumor (carcinoma *in situ*)

p^{T1} Limited to testis and epididymis

p^{T2} As pT1 and vascular/lymphatic invasion or involvement of tunica vaginalis

p^{T3} Invasion of spermatic cord

p^{T4} Invasion of scrotum

p^{N0} Negative lymph nodes

p^{N1} Node 20 mm; or 5 nodes involved all <20 mm

p^{N2} Node between 20 and 50 mm; or >5 nodes none >50 mm

p^{N3} Node mass >50 mm

M0   No distant metastasis

M1   Distant metastasis

GRADING OF VARICOCELE

Grade	Relaxed State	During Valsalva
Normal	2.2 mm	2.7 mm
Small varicocele	2.5-4.0 mm	Increase by 1.0 mm
Moderate varicocele	4.0-5.0 mm	Increase by 1.2- 1.5 mm
Large varicocele	>5.0 mm	Increase by >1.5 mm

STAGING OF BLADDER CANCER (FIG. 11.2)

Jewett-Strong	TNM	
O	T0	No tumor
	Tis	Carcinoma *in situ*
	Ta	Papillary tumor confined to mucosa
A	T1	Invasion of lamina propria
B1	T2a	Of inner half of muscle
B2	T2b	Of outer half of muscle
C	T3	Of perivesical fat
D1	T4a	Of surrounding organs (seminal vesicles, prostate, rectum)
	T4b	pelvic/abdominal wall
	N1	metastasis to single node ≤ 2 cm
	N2	metastasis to single node of 2-5 cm/in multiple nodes ≤ 5 cm
	N3	metastasis to single node > 5 cm
D2	N4	lymph node metastasis above bifurcation of common iliac arteries
	M1	distant metastasis (lung, liver, bone)

RENAL INJURY SCALE
(AMERICAN ASSOCIATION OF SURGEONS IN TRAUMA)

Grade 1: Hematuria and normal imaging findings; renal contusion; nonexpanding subcapsular hematoma

Grade 2: Laceration of cortex (<1 cm deep); nonexpanding perirenal hematoma

Grade 3: Laceration of cortex and medulla (>1 cm deep)

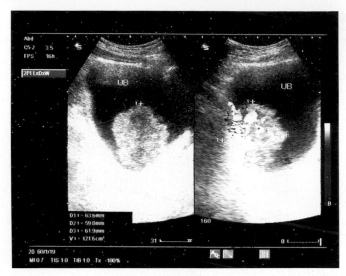

Fig. 11.2: Bladder cancer

Grade 4: (a) *Parenchymal injury:* Laceration involving
              collecting system
       (b) *Vessel injury:* Injury to renal artery/vein with
              contained hemorrhage; thrombosis of segmen-
              tal artery
Grade 5: (a) *Parenchymal injury:* Shattered kidney
       (b) *Devascularizing injury:* Avulsion/*in situ*
              thrombosis of main renal artery

GRADING OF SPLENIC INJURY

Grade	Injury	Description
I	Hematoma	Subcapsular <25% of surface area
	Laceration	Capsular tear <1 cm of parenchymal depth

II	Hematoma	Subcapsular 25-50% of surface area; intraparenchymal <5 cm in diameter
	Laceration	1-3 cm deep without involvement of trabecular vessel
III	Hematoma	Subcapsular >50% of surface area; ruptured subcapsular/parenchymal; intraparenchymal >10 cm/expanding
	Laceration	>3 cm parenchymal depth/involvement of trabecular vessels
IV	Laceration	Involving segmental/hilar vessels with devascularization of >25%
V	Laceration	Completely shattered spleen
	Vascular	Total splenic devascularization

GRADING OF LIVER INJURY

Grade	Injury	Description
I	Hematoma	Subcapsular <10% of surface area
	Laceration	Capsular tear <1 cm of parenchymal depth
II	Hematoma	Subcapsular 10-50% of surface area; intraparenchymal <10 cm in diameter
	Laceration	1-3 cm deep and <10 cm long
III	Hematoma	Subcapsular >50% of surface area; ruptured subcapsular/parenchymal; intraparenchymal >10 cm/expanding
	Laceration	>3 cm parenchymal depth
IV	Laceration	Parenchymal disruption 25-75% of lobe; 1-3 Couinaud segments in single lobe

V	Laceration	Disruption >75% of single lobe; >3 Couinaud segments in single lobe
	Vascular	Juxtahepatic venous injury (HV, IVC)
VI	Vascular	Hepatic avulsion

CONGENITAL BILIARY CYSTS (TODANI CLASSIFICATION)

I. Choledochal cyst
   IA—cystic dilatation of CBD
   IB—focal segmental dilatation of CBD
   IC—fusiform dilatation of CBD
II. Diverticulum of extrahepatic ducts—originating from CBD/CHD neck of diverticulum open/closed
III. Choledochocele
IV. Multiple segmental bile duct cysts
A—multiple intra- and extrahepatic biliary cysts and saccular dilatation of CBD
B—multiple extrahepatic biliary cysts and normal intrahepatic bile ducts
Caroli's disease: Intrahepatic biliary cysts

GALLBLADDER CARCINOMA (MODIFIED NEVIN STAGE)

I   Mucosa only (*in situ* carcinoma)
II Mucosal and muscular invasion
III Mucosa and muscularis and serosa
IV Gallbladder wall and lymph nodes
V   Hepatic/distant metastases

STAGING OF COLORECTAL CANCER

Tis   Carcinoma *in situ*
T1   Invasion of submucosa

T2   Invasion of muscularis propria
T3   Invasion of subserosa/pericolic tissue
T4   Invasion of visceral peritoneum/other organs
N1   1-3 pericolic lymph node
N2   >4 pericolic lymph node
N3   Any lymph node along course of a vascular trunk.

ESOPHAGEAL CANCER CT STAGING (MOSS)

Stage 1 Intraluminal tumor/localized wall thickening of 3 - 5 mm

Stage 2 Localized/circumferential wall thickening >5 mm

Stage 3 Contiguous spread into adjacent mediastinum (trachea, bronchi, aorta, pericardium)—loss of fat planes (nonspecific due to cachexia, often still resectable)—mass in contact with aorta >90° arc (in 20-70% still resectable)—displacement/compression of airway'- esophagotracheal/bronchial fistula (unresectable)

Stage 4 Distant metastases–enlarged abdominal lymph nodes >10 mm—hepatic, pulmonary, adrenal metastases, direct erosion of vertebral body—tumor >3 cm wide—high frequency of extraesophageal spread.

GASTRIC CARCINOMA STAGING

T1   Tumor limited to mucosa/submucosa
T2   Tumor involves muscle/serosa
T3   Tumor penetrates through serosa
T4a Invasion of adjacent contiguous tissues
T4b Invasion of adjacent organs, diaphragm, abdominal wall

N1   Involvement of perigastric nodes within 3 cm of primary along greater/lesser curvature

N2   Involvement of regional nodes >3 cm from primary along branches of celiac axis

N3   Para-aortic, hepatoduodenal, retropancreatic, mesenteric nodes

M1   Distant metastases

CLASSIFICATION OF JAPAN RESEARCH SOCIETY FOR GASTRIC CANCER

Type I   Protruded type ≥ 5 mm in height with protrusion into gastric lumen

Type II   Superficial type ≤ 5 mm in height

IIa   Slightly elevated surface

IIb   Flat/almost unrecognizable

IIc   Slightly depressed surface

Type III Excavated/ulcerated type

ADVANCED GASTRIC CANCER (T2 LESION AND HIGHER) BORMANN CLASSIFICATION

Type 1   Broad-based elevated polypoid lesion

Type 2   Elevated lesion, ulceration and well-demarcated margin

Type 3   Elevated lesion, ulceration and ill-defined margin

Type 4   Ill-defined flat lesion

Type 5   Unclassified, no apparent elevation

LYMPHOMA OF GASTROINTESTINAL TRACT

CT Staging

Stage I   Tumor confined to bowel wall

Stage II   Limited to local nodes

Stage III Widespread nodal disease
Stage IV Disseminated to bone marrow, liver, other organs

AMPULLARY TUMOR

Benign/malignant tumors arising from glandular epithelium of ampulla of Vater.

TNM Staging

T1: Tumor confined to ampulla
T2: Tumor extending into duodenal wall
T3: Invasion of pancreas <2 cm deep
T4: Invasion of pancreas >2 cm deep

AORTIC DISSECTION

DeBakey classification	Part involved
Type I	Ascending aorta and portion distal to arch
Type II	Ascending aorta only
Type III	Descending aorta only
Subtype III A	Up to diaphragm
Subtype III B	Below diaphragm

STANFORD CLASSIFICATION

Type A: Ascending aorta Â± arch in first 4 cm
Type B: Descending aorta only

TNM STAGING OF LUNG CANCER

Stage	Description
T1	<3 cm in diameter, surrounded by lung/visceral pleura.
T2	≥ 3 cm in diameter/invasion of visceral pleura/lobar atelectasis/obstructive pneumonitis/at least 2 cm from carina.
T3	Tumor of any size; less than 2 cm from carina/invasion of parietal pleura, chest wall, diaphragm, mediastinal pleura, pericardium; pleural effusion; satellite nodule in same lobe.
T4	Invasion of heart, great vessels, trachea, esophagus, vertebral body, carina/malignant pleural effusion.
N1	Peribronchial/ipsilateral hilar nodes.
N2	Ipsilateral mediastinal nodes.
N3	Contralateral hilar/mediastinal nodes, scalene/supraclavicular nodes.

CYSTIC ADENOMATOID MALFORMATION

It refers to congenital cystic abnormality of the lung, characterized by an intralobar mass of disorganized pulmonary tissue communicating with bronchial tree and having normal vascular supply, drainage but delayed clearance of fetal lung fluid.

OB-USG FINDINGS

Type I Single large cyst/multiple large cysts of 2-10 cm in diameter

Type II Multiple small cysts of 5-12 mm in diameter

Type III Large homogeneously hyperechoic mass compared with liver.

HODGKIN DISEASE

Ann Arbor Staging Classification

Stage I	Limited to one/two contiguous anatomic regions on same side of diaphragm
Stage II	>2 anatomic regions/two noncontiguous regions on same side of diaphragm
Stage III	On both sides of diaphragm, not extending beyond lymph nodes, spleen (Stage III$_S$), Waldeyer's ring
III$_E$	With extralymphatic organ/site
Stage IV	Organ involvement (bone marrow, bone, lung, pleura, liver, kidney, GI tract, skin) ± lymph node involvement
E	Extralymphatic site
S	Splenic involvement
Substage A	Absence of systemic symptoms
Substage B	Fever, night sweats, pruritus, ≥10% weight loss in past 6 months

THYROID OPHTHALMOPATHY/ GRAVE'S DISEASE OF ORBIT

Staging (Werner's modified classification)

Stage	I	Eyelid retraction without symptoms
Stage	II	Eyelid retraction with symptoms
Stage	III	Proptosis >22 mm without diplopia
Stage	IV	Proptosis >22 mm with diplopia
Stage	V	Corneal ulceration
Stage	VI	Loss of sight

MR CLASSIFICATION OF MENISCAL INJURY

Grade	Type	MR Finding
0	0	normal meniscus
1	I	globular/punctate intrameniscal signal
2	II	linear signal not extending to surface
	III	short-tapered apex of meniscus
	IV	truncated/blunted apex of meniscus
3	V	signal extending to only one surface 85%
3	VI	signal extending to both surfaces
3	VII	comminuted reticulated signal pattern

PARAOSTEOARTHROPATHY/ ECTOPIC OSSIFICATION/ MYOSITIS OSSIFICANS

Radiographic Grading System (Brooker)

0   No soft-tissue ossification
I   Separate small foci of ossification
II >1 cm gap between opposing bone surfaces of heterotopic ossifications
III <1 cm gap between opposing bone surfaces
IV Bridging ossification

ATLANTOAXIAL ROTARY FIXATION

Grading

I   <3 mm anterior displacement of atlas on axis
II 3-5 mm anterior displacement of atlas on axis
III > 5 mm anterior displacement of atlas on axis
IV Posterior displacement of atlas on axis

ASCITES

Grading

Mild—when minimal free fluid is present in morrisons pouch/pouch of Douglas

Moderate—when fluid is present in both flanks also

Severe—fluid fills the whole abdominal cavity and pelvis, Bowel loops seen floating in fluid.

Note

- 50- 75 ml of free fluid is present in the peritoneal cavity, this acts as lubricant
- Transvaginal scan is most sensitive to detect free fluid, can detect as small as 0.8 ml free fluid also.

PLEURAL EFFUSION (FIG. 11.3)

Classification: Mainly based on radiological experience—
- Mild
- Moderate
- Severe

Quantity of fluid estimation by **USG**

Measure the maximum perpendicular distance between the chest wall and the lung surface

Measurement is made above the level of diaphragm, e.g.

20 mm width = 380 ± 130 ml

40 mm width = 1000 ± 330 ml

HYDROCELE

- It refers to collection of fluid between parietal and visceral layers of tunica vaginalis.
- It is the most common cause of testicular swelling.

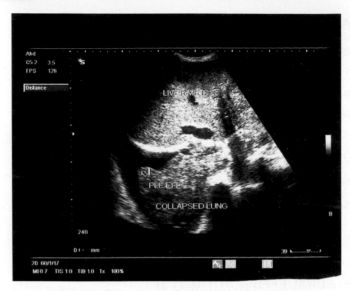

Fig. 11.3: Right pleural effusion with collapsed lung

Classification: Mainly based on radiological experience—
- *Mild*—when minimal free fluid is present both anterior and posterior to testis
- *Moderate*
- *Severe*

Types

- Congenital hydrocele
- Idiopathic hydrocele (primary)
- Secondary hydrocele

Common Causes
- Torsion
- Trauma/postsurgical

- Epididymitis, epididymoorchitis
- Testicular tumor.

SLIPPED CAPITAL FEMORAL EPIPHYSIS

Refers to atraumatic fracture through hypertrophic zone of physeal plate of femur
  Grading (based on femoral head position)
- *Mild*—displaced by <1/3 of metaphyseal diameter
- *Moderate*—displaced by 1/3 - 2/3 of diameter
- *Severe*—displaced by >2/3 of metaphyseal diameter

Common Causes

- Rickets
- Renal osteodystrophy
- Trauma
- Growth spurt.

ACROMIOCLAVICULAR DISLOCATION GRADING

Grade 1   Soft-tissue swelling and no joint widening
Grade 2   Subluxation with elevation of clavicle of <5 mm
Grade 3   Dislocation with wide AC joint and increased coracoclavicular distance

SPONDYLOLISTHESIS

It refers to displacement of one vertebra over another.
Grades I-IV (Meyerding method)—each grade equals to 1/4 anterior subluxation of upper vertebral body on lower.

Common Causes

- Fracture
- Bone tumor

- Scoliosis
- Degenerative disk disease.

Three types based on direction of displacement
- Retrolisthesis
- Anterolisthesis
- Lateral translation

Spondyloptosis—when vertebral body has slipped completely beyond the sacral promontory

SCORING SYSTEM FOR OVARIAN TUMORS

Scoring system for ovarian tumors is based on following factors:

Inner Wall Structure

Score

1. Smooth
2. Irregularities < 3 mm
3. Papillarities > 3 mm
4. Mostly solid

Wall Thickness

Score

1. Thin < 3 mm
2. Thick > 3 mm
3. Mostly solid

Septa

Score

1. Absent

2. Thin < 3 mm
3. Thick > 3 mm

Echogenicity

Score

1. Sonolucent
2. Low echogenicity
3. Low echogenicity with echogenic core
4. Mixed echogenicity
5. High echogenicity

Total Score Range: 4-15

Score Suspicious for Malignancy ≥ 9

Placenta Previa

Grading

Complete—placenta totally covers the internal os

Partial—placenta partially covers the os

Marginal- placenta extends to the edge of internal os

Low lying placenta—distance of placenta tip from internal os is < 5 cm

GRADING OF NEONATAL CEREBRAL HEMORRHAGE

Grade I—Isolated subependymal hemorrhage

Grade II—Subependymal hemorrhage with ventricular extension (< 50 % ventricular lumen)

Grade III—Intraventricular hemorrhage (> 50 % ventricular lumen) and ventricular dilation

Grade IV—Additional extension to cerebral parenchyma

Plain Abdominal Radiographic Classification of Small Bowel Obstruction

- *Normal*—when small intestine gas is absent/gas within 3-4 variably shaped loops <2.5 cm in diameter
- *Mild small bowel obstruction*—when single/multiple loops of 2.5-3 cm in diameter with ≥3 air-fluid levels
- *Probable small bowel obstruction*—when multiple dilated gas-/fluid-filled loops with air-fluid levels and moderate amount of colonic gas
- *Definite small bowel obstruction*—in this type clearly disproportionate gaseous/fluid distension of small bowel is seen relative to colon.

Graf Classification—Developmental Dysplasia of Hip (DDH)

Type I

- Good cartilaginous and osseous roofing of femoral head, normal contact and centring of femoral head.
- *Alpha angle* ≥ 60°
- *Beta angle* ≤ 55°
- Comment—normal
- Treatment—none

Type IIa

- Sufficient roofing of femoral head but poor ooseous roof
- No ossification of femoral epiphysis
- *Alpha angle*—50-60°
- *Beta angle*—55-77°
- *Comment*— < 3 months physiologically immature
- *Treatment*—observe until mature

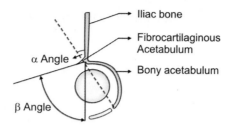

Fig. 11.4: Coronal view of right hip

α Angle—Refers to angle between bony acetabular margin and straight lateral edge of ilium

β Angle—Refers to angle between fibrocartilaginous accetabulum and straight lateral edge of ilium

Type IIb

- Sufficient roofing of femoral head but poor ooseous roof
- No ossification of femoral epiphysis
- *Alpha angle*—50-60°
- *Beta angle*—55-77°
- *Comment*—> 3 months delayed maturity
- *Treatment*—follow-up and consider abduction orthosis.

Type IIIa

- Cartilagenous roof pushed upward
- Femoral head pushed cranially subluxing
- No structural change of cartilage
- *Alpha angle* ≤ 43°
- *Beta angle* ≥ 77°
- *Comment*—cartilage normal echogenicity
- *Treatment*—reduce.

Type IIIb

- Progression of cartilaginous roof pushed upward.

- Femoral head subluxing, structural change of cartilage
- *Alpha angle* ≤ 43°
- *Beta angle* ≥ 77°
- *Comment*—cartilage increased echogenicity
- *Treatment*—reduce

Type IV

- Acetabulum empty and femoral head lying in soft tissues
- *Alpha angle*—not measurable
- *Beta angle*—not measurable
- *Comment*—very shallow
- *Treatment*—reduce, possible open reduction.

CRITERIA TO ASSESS NODAL DISEASE

Location	Classification	Size
Pelvic	Abnormal	> 1.5 cm
Retrocrural	Abnormal	> 0.6 cm
Abdomen	Normal	< 1 cm
	Suspicious	> 1 cm, single
	Abnormal	>1 cm, multiple
	Abnormal	> 1.5 cm, single

CARDIOTHORACIC RATIO

Refers to ratio of widest transverse cardiac diameter to widest inside thoracic diameter.

Grading

<0.45—normal
0.45-0.55—mild cardiomegaly

>0.55—severe cardiomegaly
< 0.5 is normal in >1 month old
< 0.6 is normal in <1 month old.

CARDIOMEGALY

Common causes are:
- Congestive heart failure
- Pericardial effusion
- Multivalvular disease
- False cardiomegaly—in supine position and expiration.

CARDIOMEGALY IN NEWBORN

Common causes are:
- Congenital heart disease
- Cardiac tumor
- Pericarditis/myocarditis
- Transient tachypnea of newborn
- Anemia
- Thyroid disease—hypo-/hyperthyroidism
- Infant of diabetic mother.

IMPERFORATE ANUS

There are three categories:
1. *High anomaly:* In this type, bowel ends above levator sling, fistulous connection to perineum/vagina/posterior urethra (air in bladder in males; air in vagina in females)
2. *Intermediate defect:* In this type, bowel ends within levator muscle as a result of abnormality in posterior migration of rectum, fistula opening low in vagina/vestibule.

3. *Low anomaly:* In this type, bowel has passed through levator sling, fistula to perineum/vulva.

Measurement Findings on USG

≤15 mm distance between anal dimple and distal rectal pouch on transperineal images indicates low anomaly.

Chapter 12

Age Determination
by Radiographs

TEETH DEVELOPMENT

Deciduous teeth	Eruption (month)	Shedding (yr)
Medial incisors	6–8	7
Lateral incisors	7–12	8
First molars	14–15	10
Canines	18–19	10
Second molars	20–24	11–12

PERMANENT TEETH

	Boys	Girls
First molars	6.5 yr	6.0 yr
Medial incisors	7.0 yr	6.5 yr
Lateral incisors	8.5 yr	8.0 yr
First premolars	10.0 yr	9.0 yr
Second premolars	11.0 yr	10.0 yr
Canines	11.5 yr	11.0 yr
Second molars	12 yr	11.5 yr
Third molars	17–25 yr	17–25 yr

CENTERS OF OSSIFICATION

Shoulder Joint

Secondary center	Appear
Head of humerus	1 yr
Greater tuberosity	3 yr
Lesser tuberosity	5 yr

These three centers unite at 6 years and form conjoint epiphysis and fuse shaft by 20 years

Secondary center	Appear	Fuse by
Two epiphysis for acromion	15–18 yr	25 yr
Middle of coracoid process	1 yr	15 yr
Root of coracoid process	17 yr	25 yr
Inferior angle of scapula	14–20 yr	22–25 yr
Medial border of scapula	14–20 yr	22–25 yr
Sternal end of clavicle	18–20 yr	25 yr

ELBOW JOINT

Secondary center	Appear	Fuse by
Capitulum	1–3 yr	17–18 yr
Head of radius	5–6 yr	16–19 yr
Internal epicondyle	5–8 yr	17–18 yr
External epicondyle	10–12 yr	17–18 yr
Trochlea	11 yr	18 yr
Olecranon	10–13 yr	16–20 yr

HAND WITH WRIST JOINT

Secondary center	Appear	Fuse by
Lower end of radius	1–2 yr	20 yr
Lower end of ulna	5–8 yr	20 yr
Metacarpal heads	2 yr 6 m	20 yr
Base of proximal phalanges	2 yr 6m	20 yr
Base of middle phalanges	3 yr	18–20 yr
Base of distal phalanges	3 yr	18–20 yr
Base of first metacarpal	2 yr 6 m	20 yr

Primary center	*Appear*
Capitate	4 m
Hamate	4 m
Triquetral	3 yr
Lunate	4–5 yr
Trapezium	6 yr
Trapezoid	6 yr
Scaphoid	6 yr
Pisiform	11 yr

Chapter 13

Rules in
Radiology

SCAN WHERE IT HURTS

According to this rule during sonography focus more on the part where patient is having more tenderness.

For example,

Sonographic Murphy sign—in cholecystitis

Sonographic McBurney sign—in appendicitis.

RULE OF TENS (TEN% TUMOR)

Pheochromocytoma follows it:

10% bilateral/multiple

10% familial

10% malignant

10% extra-adrenal

10 % of insulinoma:

10% are associated with men 1

10% are multiple

10% have islet cell hyperplasia

10% are malignant.

Rule of 10'S

Wilms' tumor follows it:

- 10% unfavorable histology
- 10% bilateral
- 10% vascular invasion
- 10% calcifications
- 10% pulmonary metastases at presentation.

Rule of Three's

Spinal cord follows it, above L3 by age 3 months, i.e. spinal cord should be above L3 vertebrae by age of 3 months.

Abnormality: Tethered cord/Tight filum terminale Syndrome/ Low conus medullaris.

It refers to abnormally short and thickened filum terminale with position of conus medullaris below L2-3.

Rule of 3's

Small bowel follows it:
- Wall thickness <3 mm
- Valvulae conniventes <3 mm
- Diameter <3 cm
- Air-fluid levels <3.

Rule of 3's

Hydrostatic/pneumatic reduction follows it:
- *Indication:* Intussusception
- *CID:* Peritonitis, pneumoperitoneum, hypovolemic shock.

Procedure

- Patient is sedated
- Anal seal is put with 24-F Foley's catheter and balloon inflated; balloon pulled down to levator sling; taped to buttocks; and both buttocks firmly taped together.
- Air or 60% wt/vol barium sulfate with container between 24-36 inches above level of anus:
  - 3.5 feet (105 cm) above table
  - 3 attempts max
  - 3 minutes between attempts (delay allows venous congestion and edema to subside).

Rule of 1/3

Carcinoid follows it:
- 1/3 occur in small bowel

- 1/3 have metastases
- 1/3 are multiple
- 1/3 have a second malignancy.

RULE OF 2s

Meckel's diverticulum follows it:
- This diverticulum is formed due to persistence of the Vitelline duct, which usually obliterates by 5th embryonic week
- Common in 2% of population, symptomatic usually before age of 2 years, located within 2 feet of ileocecal valve, length of 2 inches.

4711 RULE

It refers to normal splenic measurements:
- Thickness   — 4 cm
- A-P diameter— 7 cm
- Length   — 11cm

Most commonly used method is:
Eyeball technique, i.e. if it looks big, it is Big.

Rule of Thumb

Crown-rump length (CRL) follows it. It refers to the length of fetus.
- Menstrual age in weeks = CRL (in cm) + 6

Renal Measurements

As a rule left kidney is usually 2% longer than right kidney.

As a rule, normally:
- Left hilum is at higher level than right hilum
- Right dome of diaphragm is at higher level than left dome
- Left kidney is at higher level than right kidney
- Right testis is at higher level than left testis.

Rule of Eight

Applied in case of delayed contrast excretion by kidneys in IVU study. For example: If it takes 30 minutes for contrast to fill the calices, then 4 hours is about right for the next film and so on (i.e. next film is taken 8 times of first).

Harris Rule of 12s

- This is applied to diagnose atlanto-occipital dislocation
- In this two distances are measured:
  - Distance from the base of dens to the clivus
  - Distance from a line drawn from the posterior wall of dens to the clivus.
- Considered abnormal if clivus is >12 mm above the tip of dens or 12 mm anterior to the posterior dens line.

Ten Days Rule

According to this rule diagnostic X-ray irradiation procedure involving the pelvic region of females of child bearing age shall be limited to the 10 days period, following the onset of last menstruation, in order to prevent irradiation of an unrecognized early pregnancy.

Portosystemic Venous Collaterals Rule

According to this rule presence of portosystemic collaterals is a clear indication of portal hypertension. Except in case of collaterals related to isolated splenic or mesentric vein occlusion.

Venous Distention Rule

According to this rule, recently thrombosed veins are generally distended to an abnormal large size and are substantially larger than the adjacent artery except if thrombus is small and non-occlusive or if the vein is scarred and is incapable of dilation.

Chapter 14

Hounsfield Unit Values

		HU value
Air	-	-1000
Lung	-	$-700 +/- 200$
Fat	-	$-90 +/10$
Fat/connective tissue	-	$-15 +/- 65$
Spongy bone	-	$130 +/- 100$
Compact bone	-	> 250
Water	-	$0 +/- 5$

PARENCHYMAL ORGANS 50 +/– 40

		HU value
Suprarenal gland	-	$17 +/- 7$
Transudate	-	$18 +/- 2$
Effusion/exudate	-	$25 +/- 5$
Kidney	-	$30 +/- 10$
Pancreas	-	$40 +/- 10$
Spleen/Lymphoma/Muscle	-	$45 +/- 5$
A/c hemorrhage	-	$55 +/- 5$
Liver	-	$65 +/- 5$
Thyroid	-	$70 +/- 10$
Clotted blood	-	$80 +/- 10$
CSF	-	≤ 10

Chapter 15

Basics of MRI

BASICS OF MRI SIGNALS

Dark Signal on T1-WI

- Flow void
- Increased water as in hemorrhage (hyperacute or chronic), tumor, edema, infarction, infection, inflammation.
- Calcification.

Dark Signal on T2-WI

- Flow void
- Protein-rich fluid
- Paramagnetic substances: Deoxyhemoglobin, iron, ferritin, intracellular methemoglobin, melanin, hemosiderin
- Fibrous tissue, calcification.

Bright Signal on T1-WI

- Fat
- Melanin
- Protein-rich fluid
- Subacute hemorrhage
- Slowly flowing blood
- Laminar necrosis of cerebral infarction
- Paramagnetic substances: Manganese, gadolinium, copper.

Bright Signal on T2-WI

- Increased water as in tumor, edema, infarction, infection, inflammation, subdural collection
- Extracellular methemoglobin in subacute hemorrhage.

MR SPECTROSCOPY

Spectral Peaks

1. *Amino acids:*
   - Alanine - Peak is between 1.3 and 1.5 ppm
     - Increased levels seen commonly in meningiomas.
   - Leucine [3.6 ppm] and valine [0.9 ppm]-these are key markers of abscesses.
2. *Lipids:*
   - These produce multiple resonances, important peaks are at 0.8 to 0.9 and 1.2 to 1.3 ppm.
   - Increased levels seen in meningiomas, high grade gliomas, lymphomas, necrotic foci, demyelination and inborn errors of metabolism.
3. *Lactate:*
   - It is identified as a doublet peak [as it splits into 2 separate peaks, separated by 0.2 ppm] centered at 1.32 ppm
   - It is an indicator of anaerobic glycolysis due to seizure neoplasms, hypoxia, infarcts, and metabolic disorders
4. *NAA:*
   - Peak occurs at 2.02 ppm.
   - Decreased levels seen in neurodegenerative diseases, tumors, stroke, multiple sclerosis.and epilepsy
   - Increased levels seen in Canavan's disease.
5. *Glutamine, Glutamate, Gabu:*
   - These are a complex set of resonances at 2.1 and 2.5 ppm.
   - This peak complex is noted in schizophrenia and epilepsy.

6. *Creatinine:*
   - Peak occurs at 3.02 ppm.
   - Decreased levels seen in brain tumours particularly malignant.
7. *Choline:*
   - Peak occurs at at 3.2 ppm.
   - Decreased levels seen in hypomyelinating diseases
   - Increased levels seen in primary brain tumors and demyelinating diseases.
8. *Myoinositol:*
   - It produces two peaks but forms major component at 3.56 ppm.
   - Decreased levels seen in hepatic encephalopathy and hyponatremia.
   - Increased levels seen in demyelinating diseases and Alzheimer's disease, chronic HIE.

Bibliography

- Grainger and Allison. Diagnostic Radiology.
- David Sutton. Textbook of Radiology and Imaging.
- Wolf Gang Dahnert. Radiology Review Manual.
- Carol M Rumack. Diagnostic Ultrasound.
- Theodore E Keats. Atlas of Radiologic Measurement.
- Yochum Rowe. Essentials of Skeletal Radiology.
- Osborn. Diagnostic Imaging Brain.
- Mathias Hofer. CT Teaching Manual.
- Mathias Hofer. Ultrasound Teaching Manual.
- Palmer. Manual of Diagnostic Ultrasound.
- Lee Sagel, Stanley Huken. Computed Body Tomography with MRI Correlation.

Index